THE MEDICINE CHEST

THE MEDICINE CHEST

A Physician's Journey towards Reconciliation

JAROL BOAN

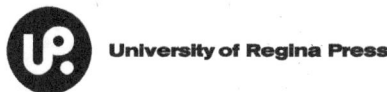
University of Regina Press

Copyright © 2024 Jarol Boan

All rights reserved. No part of this work covered by the copyrights hereon may be reproduced or used in any form or by any means—graphic, electronic, or mechanical—without the prior written permission of the publisher. Any request for photocopying, recording, taping, or placement in information storage and retrieval systems of any sort shall be directed in writing to Access Copyright.

Printed and bound in Canada. The text of this book is printed on 100% post-consumer recycled paper with earth-friendly vegetable-based inks.

Cover art: "First Aid Kit" by krasyuk / AdobeStock
Cover design: Duncan Noel Campbell, University of Regina Press
Interior layout design: John van der Woude, JVDW Designs
Copyeditor: Rachel Ironstone
Proofreader: Crissy Calhoun
Indexer: François Trahan

Library and Archives Canada Cataloguing in Publication

Title: The medicine chest : a physician's journey towards reconciliation / Jarol Boan.
Names: Boan, Jarol, author.
Description: Includes index.
Identifiers: Canadiana (print) 20230553281 | Canadiana (ebook) 20230553478 | ISBN 9780889779761 (hardcover) | ISBN 9780889779730 (softcover) | ISBN 9780889779747 (PDF) | ISBN 9780889779754 (EPUB)
Subjects: LCSH: Indigenous peoples—Health and hygiene—Canada. | LCSH: Indigenous peoples—Medical care—Canada. | LCSH: Discrimination in medical care—Canada. | LCSH: Health services accessibility—Canada.
Classification: LCC RA450.4.I53 B63 2024 | DDC 362.1089/97071—dc23

10 9 8 7 6 5 4 3 2 1

University of Regina Press, University of Regina
Regina, Saskatchewan, Canada, S4S 0A2
TEL: (306) 585-4758 FAX: (306) 585-4699
WEB: www.uofrpress.ca

U OF R PRESS

We acknowledge the support of the Canada Council for the Arts for our publishing program. We acknowledge the financial support of the Government of Canada. Nous reconnaissons l'appui financier du gouvernement du Canada. This publication was made possible with support from Creative Saskatchewan's Book Publishing Production Grant program.

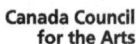 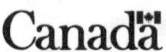

*To Val Desjarlais (1959–2021)
for her dedication to saving Indigenous lives*

CONTENTS

Acknowledgements ix
Map xi

Introduction xiii

Willow Medicine 1
Hollywood in Regina 7
A Field on the Prairie 25
A Middle Ground 33
Two-Eyed Seeing 43
A Crime to Refuse Treatment 55
As Long as That Sun Shines 67
Strangers in the Touchwood Hills 75
An Expanding Circle 83
Red Dress Day 99
Michael's Tears 111
An HIV Epidemic 121
A Clinic in the Parklands 129
Derrick 139
The Trade in Alcohol 149
Maybe I Will, Maybe I Won't 163
Sweetgrass and Ceremony 175

The Dialysis Shuttle   189
Anxiety   203
Food on the Reserve   221
The Spirit Journey   233
Ten to Fifteen Percent   241
The Serpent   251
The Road to Reconciliation   271

Seven Grandfather Teachings from the Anishinaabe   281
Postscript   283
TRC Calls to Action addressed in *The Medicine Chest*   287

Index   289
About the Author   307

ACKNOWLEDGEMENTS

I want to thank my patients and their families for expanding and enriching my knowledge of medicine. My appreciation also goes to the leaders and officials on the reserves who have welcomed me and to my colleagues in the Wellness Wheel project and in the hospitals of Regina, Saskatchewan. A special thanks is directed to those who have helped me to shape this book and to look for a compassionate and respectful approach. My apologies are offered to anyone who feels that I have not met this standard.

I would also like to thank the following people who provided insights as I have struggled on my journey: Tanyss Knowles, Ian McLeod, Stu Skinner, Susanne Nicolay, JoLee Sasakamoose, Blair Stonechild, Jeffie Anderson, Karen Palmer, Swapna Deshpande, Simone Hengen, Lesley Cameron, Alex Wong, David Kopriva, Patrick Duffy, Michelle Archer, Roxanne Wagner, Carol Longman and family, Cynthia Kay, Ibriam Khan, Trevor Herriot, Peter Pratt, Joyce Pratt, Stan Bird, Dexter Asapace, the family of Irvin and Doris Buffalo, Max Itittakoose, Sarah Lisowitch, Rachel Asiniwasis, Thanh Luu, Megan Clark, Keiran Conway, Vicki Schultz, Maria Campbell, Eleanor Sunshine, Brian Gellor, Greg Marchildon, Carla Crozier, Stephanie Konrad, Noreen Reed, Connie Walker, Dean Bellegarde, and Doug Stewart.

Thank you to the staff at University of Regina Press for believing in this work and shepherding these words into a final product. They have provided endless encouragement, technical skills, valuable insights, and enthusiasm.

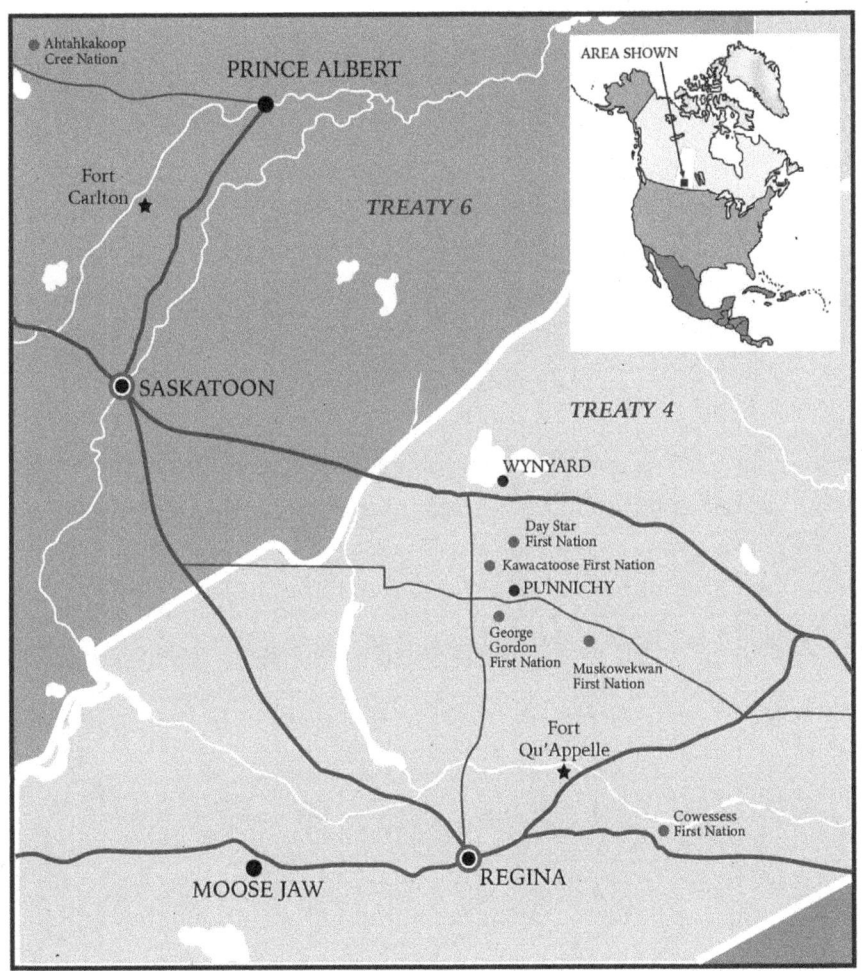

Region of Saskatchewan covered in the book. *Map by Cindy Farnsworth, 2022.*

INTRODUCTION

I want first to acknowledge that I have written this account while living and working in Treaty 4 and Treaty 6 lands, the traditional lands of the nêhiyawak, Anihšināpēk, Dakota, Lakota, and Nakoda, and in the homeland of the Métis/Michif Nation. I pay my respects to the traditional caretakers of this land.

In these chapters, I share my experience of working with Indigenous patients and their families within the Saskatchewan health care system since 2011. Except where noted, I have avoided the use of real names in my descriptions of patients and families. My portraits of individual patients have been built from multiple experiences with the illnesses and conditions that I describe. Those whose names I have mentioned have given me permission to do so.

The oppression of Indigenous people is entrenched in Canada's health care system, as it is in other institutions. As I was working on this book, Canadian media carried regular and disturbing reports about racism in health care: a man who died in a Winnipeg hospital waiting room for lack of care; a woman in Quebec who was mocked by nurses in her last moments of life. An Indigenous physician posted an article recalling how she had saved her father's life as a medical student when she rescued him from an ER team that refused to give him medication. They assumed he was an abuser of street drugs and "they didn't know what he was on."

I grew up in Regina, Saskatchewan, where much of this book is set. However, I spent thirty years of my career as a physician in other places, mostly practising and teaching in the United States. Upon returning to my hometown at the age of fifty-seven I saw that Indigenous people played a different role in Saskatchewan's affairs than they once had. They had grown in numbers, presence, and political power. My reaction to these changes was to begin to recognize, more than ever, the profound inequalities and injustices that Indigenous people face. I have gone through a long unsettling process of awakening to this obvious fact, and I am still growing. The COVID-19 pandemic, and its particular effects on Indigenous communities, has accelerated this awakening.

My approach to medical care has evolved. I am impatient with the view that the doctor's role is to prescribe pills and hope for the best. With developing optimism I see that a significant cohort of my physician colleagues, young and old, are searching for a different model of care. Social conditions are among the key determinants of health; to be effective, physicians should be part of a team that includes nurses, social workers, administrators, and other non-clinical professionals, all charged with helping the patient navigate their social environment and deal with the impacts. More and more, since my return to Canada, I have shifted my professional focus to outreach work in the rural and Indigenous communities of Saskatchewan.

Terminology is challenging in Canada, especially in the context of communities who have lost their traditional land base. In the United States, with a different social and legal history, "American Indian" or "Native American" are accepted terms. Within Canada, there are several ways that Indigenous people self-identify—one based in law and legislation, and the other within communities. The legal government definition came about in 1876 when the Indian Act codified "status" and "non-status" people. Having a status card implies a formal relationship with the Government of Canada in terms of taxation, social benefits, and health care benefits. At the time of treaty signing, many Indigenous nations were moved onto reserves and were considered "Treaty Indians." This term is now outdated. In many parts of Canada, many Indigenous people did not sign treaties, yet they have status cards. Furthermore, the Constitution Act of 1982, Section 35(2), defined three groups of Aboriginal people in Canada as First Nations, Métis, and Inuit. First Nations referred to Indigenous people who are distinct from Métis or Inuit. Then in 2014, through legal challenges, the Daniels decision determined (for certain government purposes) that Métis people were "Indians." I have used the term "Indigenous" throughout this book where possible, which is a more inclusive term.

These definitions do not define the specific cultural and linguistic traditions of those whose family roots were from mixed ancestry (intermarrying within clans or with Europeans). Nor do they describe how Indigenous people define themselves. It is my observation that Indigenous people define themselves within a particular family, clan, or nation. First Nations or community is occasionally used to describe some communities who define themselves by identifiers such as band, nation, or language.

With regard to the use of the term "Indian" in the book, admittedly, it has derogatory connotations when used by non-Indigenous people and may have unfavourable connotations for some readers. It is sometimes used in direct quotes from interviews or to describe a racial slur, for example the myth of the drunk Indian. On a personal note, I have observed that Indigenous folk use the term freely among each other, and sometimes to tease me. After I kept one of my Indigenous patients waiting in clinic, she jokingly accused me of "working on Indian time." I ask the reader to consider the context when the word "Indian" appears in the text.

My time spent in learning about two-eyed seeing and traditional culture through my relationships with the Touchwood Agency Tribal

Council and other Indigenous communities brought me into treaty[1] with the land and the Indigenous Peoples of Turtle Island. I come from a settler family with many different relations I want to honour. I want to stand in solidarity with my settler and Indigenous contemporaries and to continue to learn about colonial history to inform a more honest understanding of Canada—a reality that recognizes the cultural devastation inflicted by the settlement of the prairies under the British Crown, and the hope that healing our relationship will in turn heal our bodies, spirits, and land. To all my patients who have been my teachers, I say thank you, chi miigwetch.

Mitakuye oyasin, we are all related.

---

[1] "The Treaties were based on First Nations principles: (1) 'Myowîcêhtowin' ('Getting along with others'); (2) 'Wîtaskêwin' ('Living together on the land'); and (3) 'Pimâcihowin' ('Making a living'). Treaties were to provide both sides with the means of achieving survival and socio-economic stability, anchored on the principle of mutual benefit." From Office of the Treaty Commissioner, *Treaty Essential Learnings: We Are All Treaty People* (Saskatoon: Office of the Treaty Commissioner, 2008), 9, http://www.otc.ca/resource/purchase/treaty_essential_learnings_we_are_all_treaty_people.html?page=3.

WILLOW MEDICINE

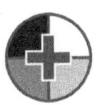

Imagine an Elder tells me a story. We are in my office, located on a busy street in Regina. I am sitting at a desk behind a laptop computer, and he is resting in an armchair at the side of the room. Despite his age, he's lean and athletic. His name is John Morris, and he needs medicine for joint pain. We have finished our clinical visit, and now he wants to tell me about his name. I push the laptop aside and lean back to listen.

Turtle Island is the term that many Indigenous people use for the continent that settlers call North America. The term originated in Saskatchewan territory, John says, because the land was flat, warm, and dry, and the turtle could find a warm place to rest in the sun. The turtle crawled out of the North Saskatchewan River and basked on the riverbank. The people who lived in the bush came to see the turtle, and the turtle spoke to them. The turtle predicted that pale faces would come to capture the people, and they needed to be careful. The pale faces would not understand the Medicine Wheel of land, spirit, weather, and water. They would try to trick the people into new ways of doing things. The people and the land itself would suffer.

Having spoken, the turtle slid back into the river and swam away.

Ahtahkakoop was a great leader who believed in the turtle's vision. He was called with other leaders to Fort Carlton, built on the banks of the river, to negotiate with the pale faces. The chief of the pale faces was named Commissioner Alexander Morris. He had come at the behest of the Queen of England to fulfill the British Crown's commitment to negotiate treaties with First Nations people to obtain rights for settlers to occupy the land. Morris held up a long white piece of paper with written words on it. Chief Ahtahkakoop did not read English. The agreement was finalized in oral tradition. They smoked a ceremonial pipe together.

As they smoked, Commissioner Morris listened to Chief Ahtahkakoop. By 1876, when this conversation took place, the fur trade had dwindled, and the buffalo were almost gone. Chief Ahtahkakoop saw his people starving and getting sick. As a good leader, he wanted the people to have the same medical care that white settlers had. He had observed that the travelling doctors carried a box on horseback. They administered medicines from this box, and the medicines had power. Chief Ahtahtakoop wanted this box for his people—they called it the medicine chest.

Commissioner Morris took his quill pen and bottle of ink and carefully wrote a new clause on the long piece of paper. It said, "and that a medicine chest shall be kept at the house of each Indian Agent for the use and benefit of the Indians."[1]

Chief Ahtahkakoop signed the piece of paper, known to history as Treaty 6. They smoked another prayer pipe among everyone present, seated in a circle.

Ahtahkakoop's people continued to hunt, fish, and trap on their lands. Then the settlers arrived and encroached on them. They put up

---

[1] Alexander H.G. Paterson, "The Medicine Chest," *Alberta Doctors' Digest*, July–August 2018, https://add.albertadoctors.org/issues/july-august-2018/medicine-chest/.

fences. The piece of paper, it seems, stated that Ahtahkakoop's people had given up the land. All the Indians along the river were now required to obey the terms of the treaty. The small parcels where they were confined under the treaty were called reserves. The queen appointed an Indian agent to show the Indians how to farm and raise fences.

The Indian agent arrived, and he recognized starvation among the people. He knew the settlers around the reserves needed labourers for their farms and to build their roads. The Indians could earn money for food if they left the reserve, but they needed permission from the agent, a written pass to allow the Indians to be employed off the reserve. The agent did not give a pass to everyone, just the people he liked.

The Elder has paused in his story. I sit quietly. The story is not yet done. I do not move or speak. This silence is part of the story. There are tears standing in his eyes. We both grieve the pain of starvation, illness, loss of land, loss of traditional ways. My heart aches with shame. I am white, and my white forefathers shared in the responsibility for this pain.

He continues. "My grandfather had an Indian name: Run with the Wind. The Indian agent liked my grandfather, and he knew that an Indian name would not be accepted by the settlers. He wanted to help my father and his family survive. The settlers were more likely to trust someone with a British name. The agent gave my grandfather a new name, and then he issued the pass.

"When he took that pass, my grandfather didn't know he was named after the white official who signed Treaty 6 with Ahtahkakoop. It was years later that we learned that Morris was meant to be a name that the settlers would respect. My grandfather survived and became a leader for his people in the Touchwood Hills, but the loss of our Indian names is painful."

The Elder's story finished, I write a prescription for an anti-inflammatory for his joint pain. I am required to use his legal name for the prescription because that is the name on his Saskatchewan health card. I write it knowing that this name carries a legacy of trickery.

The medicine I give him has a history based in treatments derived from willows,[2] like the trees that grow along the river where the turtle basked in the sun. Scientists have modified the acid that comes from willow trees and made it specific for the inflammatory cytokines that cause pain. Pharmaceutical companies market this medicine to doctors. The cost is covered by the benefits listed under Canada's Indian Act. John Morris, my patient, will not be required to pay for his pills. The pill that I prescribe was not in the medicine chest that the travelling doctors carried in 1876 because it had not yet been "invented." But the Indigenous people knew long before Western medicine produced aspirin that the bark from the willow tree could relieve pain. Only now is ibuprofen, a derivative of aspirin, part of the modern medicine chest that Ahtahkakoop negotiated with Alexander Morris.[3]

I am one of the keepers of the medicine chest. On a good day, I am able to provide treatment or advice that will help someone live a longer, healthier life. Over decades of loss and betrayal for Indigenous people, the medicine chest has often been empty or filled with horrors. I

---

2   Willow leaves and bark contain a substance known as salicin, which in the body can be converted to salicylic acid. Joe Schwarcz, "Forget the Willow Bark Extract—Go for Aspirin," McGill University: Office for Science and Society, September 28, 2022, https://www.mcgill.ca/oss/article/medical-history/forget-willow-bark-extract-go-aspirin.

3   When it was discovered in the mid-nineteenth century that salicylates were the active components of willow sap it allowed these compounds to be synthesized; from this, acetyl-salicylic acid, or aspirin, was developed. Likewise, chemical advances in the nineteenth through twentieth centuries led to the development of non-steroidal anti-inflammatory drugs (NSAIDs) (most of which were initially organic acids, but later non-acidic compounds were discovered). K.D. Rainsford, "Anti-Inflammatory Drugs in the 21st Century," *Inflammation in the Pathogenesis of Inflammatory Diseases* (Volume 42 in the Subcellular Biochemistry series, 2007), 3–27, https://doi.org/10.1007/1-4020-5688-5_1.

was unaware of this complexity when I returned to Saskatchewan in 2011, full of idealism and determined to build shared understanding and respect. Today, settler physicians like me struggle to achieve even a degree of trust with our patients.

HOLLYWOOD IN REGINA

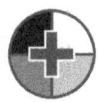

I flew to Regina from Pennsylvania, with a stopover in Minneapolis, in August 2011. I showed my Canadian passport to the customs agents. My father was waiting for me. I loaded several large suitcases and my laptop computer into the trunk of his twenty-year-old car. As we drove through the city, I felt a comfortable sense of familiarity; it was like putting on a treasured but reliable coat that looked a little tattered but was still wearable.

Southern Saskatchewan is where I belong. It took me three decades of living in other places—North Carolina, Quebec, British Columbia, Pennsylvania—to discover this. I find peace in the wide prairie landscapes and the endless open blue skies. The expansiveness brings a feeling of spirituality that connects me to a greater force in the universe. I absorbed this feeling as a child, before I was taught about galaxies or God or other spiritual labels. At that point in my life, I lived in the present without a care in the world.

When the first white surveyors arrived, the site where Regina later grew up was called Pile of Bones, a rough translation of a Cree phrase the settlers heard as "wascana." Common lore has it that during the

1870s a great mound of bones had accumulated north of Wascana Creek in the last great buffalo kill. The first townsite, given the Latin name Regina, meaning "queen," to honour the British monarch Queen Victoria, was established just to the east in 1882.

When my family moved to Regina in the 1960s, the buffalo bones were long gone, ground up for fertilizer. They had been replaced by a cityscape of low-rise office buildings and wide paved streets. It was a slow-paced city, where farmers arrived in half-ton trucks to load up on lumber and seed. The green space around the provincial legislative building in Wascana Park was largely undeveloped. Our suburban bungalow lay on the edge of the prairie with a view of the open fields. My younger brothers and I hopped the fence to play with other neighbourhood children in the wheat fields. Mothers didn't work outside the home—at noon, we walked to them from school for homemade lunches—and the street was a playground. It was safe, except for mosquitos and sunburns.

In the summer of my return, I learned that Regina had changed again. It had grown up, just as I had. The wispy, fragile trees from my childhood had become tall and sturdy, providing a canopy over the house and street. Without moving, our bungalow was now closer to the centre of town, with miles of newer homes extending across the prairie of my childhood. Wascana Park had developed walking paths, picnic tables, and a marina with a restaurant. Thanks to a grant in the 1980s from the Devonian Foundation, an offshoot of Canada's Calgary-based oil industry, cycling pathways connected all edges of the expanded city. The University of Regina had new buildings and a student population of thirteen thousand. Big box stores had mushroomed along the highway approaches to town, and the economy had diversified from wheat farming to gas fracking, petroleum refining, and potash mining.

While growing up in this city, I can't remember ever seeing an Indigenous person. On my return to the city, as my father drove us home from the airport, he braked for a middle-aged woman pushing a shopping cart filled with large black plastic bags. With newcomer eyes, I observed that she was Indigenous, dressed in tight jeans, a T-shirt with *Expos* emblazoned on the front in memory of a defunct Montreal baseball team, and a straw sun hat; she had on no shoes, and her feet were dark with dirt. I wondered where she was going with her possessions. I was surprised that my father did not comment about the woman—for him the change in demographics over the last twenty-five years had happened slowly and appeared normal. He talked on, telling me how many activities he had planned for the next week: weekly morning coffee group, finance committee meeting for the Regina Early Learning Centre, lunch with a retired colleague. It seemed like his life had gotten busier since he retired.

"I'll be fine, Dad, no need to take care of me. I'm here to take care of you." Though he looked and acted seventy-five years old, he *was* ninety-four after all; despite his vibrant energy, I was aware of his age. With my medical experience in the healthy elderly, I knew that his status could change on a dime. I had realized, after my mother died, that he was living by himself and I could be helpful. Rather than get my own house or apartment, we agreed that I would move in with him, back into our family bungalow, into my childhood bedroom. As our relationship strengthened over the next seven years, he was a source of advice and support for me in navigating the politics of the Canadian health care system. We took care of each other until his death at the age of almost 101.

On the day after my arrival, I went to the hospital, located in Regina's old east side, to obtain a name badge and set up an account as a member of the Regina General Hospital staff. They asked me where my outpatient office would be located so they could send mail to my office. My *what*? I needed an office, fast! I was excited to imagine a place where I could hang up my degrees and prove to the world that I am a doctor. On the advice of an administrative worker in the hospital, I drove—in the car I had borrowed from my dad—to a three-floor brick office building at the corner of Albert Street and 12th Avenue, in the somewhat gentrified, somewhat threadbare zone just west of the city's downtown. After parking in a visitors spot, I entered a glass double door labeled *Regina Medical Centre* with several doctors' names added below. I introduced myself to Joan Cluff, the office manager, and we talked business. I liked her immediately. She offered me a transition rate to rent office space and pay for staff as I got settled into my practice in Regina.

The process was strange for me. For twenty years, through several jobs, I had held a salaried position as a general internist in the United States—faculty member at a university medical school, employee of a hospital, executive with a pharmaceutical company, advisor to national organizations. As a general internist, I am a specialist in internal medicine, with a detailed knowledge of the body's organs and circulatory systems. Internists are trained in the skill of putting complex, seemingly unrelated medical complaints into a pattern and coming up with a diagnosis and treatment plan. Now I was associate professor of medicine at the College of Medicine at the University of Saskatchewan. Having not practised in Canada before, I didn't know anything about fee-for-service medicine, the primary way that Canadian physicians are paid.

In the 1990s the job I had enjoyed most was with an FQHC, a Federally Qualified Health Center, funded by the US government to serve vulnerable populations. The government awarded grants for the employment of a team to provide health care to the uninsured in inner cities or rural areas. The premise was that by providing health care to vulnerable populations, the government would reduce costs for private hospitals with Emergency Rooms. The grants came with strings attached: patients would be charged a fee, but only up to a limited percentage of their income, and doctors would accept a salary. I was given the title of medical director at a new clinic in a city in Indiana.

Prior to my arrival at the FQHC, a community group had converted an old building to a drop-in health centre in the inner city. They had developed a harm reduction clinic for people who used drugs; a pharmacy with donated medications for diabetes, heart disease, hypertension, and infections; a debt counselling service; a housing service office; and a psychological counsellor. All of these were operated by volunteers, creating the foundation for a successful application to the federal government for FQHC status.

My salary was modest. For me, the job was fulfilling because of the people I met. My patients were lower-middle class or living in poverty. They paid their rent, but often for substandard accommodations. They struggled to find child care. They paid their electricity bills. They did not have mobile phones. They did not have internet. They worked as casual labourers or in part-time service positions, sometimes holding down two jobs. They were single moms or dads. A few were homeless, but street smart and capable of managing adversity. Nobody had extra money at the end of the month to pay for health insurance, but now with the FQHC they had medical treatment.

Later, as a doctor in Saskatchewan, an acquaintance who was having trouble paying her bills accused me of not knowing what it was like to be poor. I reflected on this and on the stereotype that every doctor lives a life of wealth and ease.

Although it was true that I always had a roof over my head and a career that gave me financial independence, I have known lean times, struggling through the first half of my career to find a level of financial security. In my salaried jobs as a doctor in the United States, the working conditions were often difficult. We had no set hours of work and no right to claim paid overtime. The doctors' schedules depended on the corporate culture of the institution. If other doctors arrived to work at 7:30 a.m., you would arrive at 7:30 a.m. If eight hours elapsed and there was still work to do because a patient had developed complications, you stayed late.

Some of my colleagues were slap-dash quick with patients and expert at running out the door. Others were diligent and thorough. When you have a system where the doctors are paid a salary, you get a bell curve of working styles. I always assumed that the reason that I was part of the stay-later group was because I was not as smart as my colleagues that left early. I assumed that they got the diagnosis quicker than I did and were more efficient. The result was that I worked even harder, staying longer to answer questions from those who sat at the bedside of their hospitalized family member, and earned less per hour than my colleagues.

My resentful acquaintance who believed I didn't know what it was like to be poor was not aware that I went through a period when I had crippling bills to pay. I had attended the University of Saskatchewan when medical school fees were very low, and I had supportive parents who helped with living expenses, so it was not a question of student debt. Though the picture has changed at Canadian medical schools since 1990, and young doctors are left with very large student loans to pay off, for me it was not a student debt—nor was it a mortgage or a payment on a high-end car. A large part of my monthly salary was going to legal bills.

I was going through a difficult divorce in the late 1990s. My husband applied for full custody of our only child, our daughter, and fought hard to remove me from her life. I did not think this was fair, and I fought back just as hard. It turned into something that lawyers call conflicted custody, resulting in many hours of court proceedings and fat legal fees—$50,000 or more. We finally got a judgment from the court for joint custody, but the debt remained.

When I took a job on medical staff at the University of North Carolina at Chapel Hill, I started with a salary that just covered a mortgage, day care, and living expenses. To pay off my legal debt, I was living from cheque to cheque and juggling my monthly credit card payments.

One summer evening, the head of my department in Chapel Hill invited me to a barbecue at his home. I felt that I had to say yes to his generous invitation. Having been brought up to bring a small gift to a party, I asked my boss if I could bring something. I was hoping he would say no. Instead, he requested a package of veggie hot dogs, for the vegetarian guests at the party. It was the end of the month, and I had five dollars to my name until I got paid. The gas gauge in my fifteen-year-old car showed almost empty. I had no money to buy hot dogs. I had a choice: go to the gas station and put five dollars in the tank so I could attend the party, or buy veggie dogs but not attend the party at all. I arrived at the party carrying nothing but a lie: I told my boss that I had forgotten about his request.

Looking back now, I am embarrassed that I lied, and I was ashamed at the time. I had always expected that my privilege as a doctor would make me immune from financial struggles. As it happened, my position as a female—albeit a white, middle-class, privileged female—in a male-dominated profession, fighting for custody of my child, had turned me into a liar by necessity at this moment in my career.

Decades later, I have a savings account with money in it. I have a wonderful relationship with my daughter. I survived a bleak period of my life. I still don't feel good about lying. I do understand, just a bit, how financial struggles can make you do things you are not proud of.

In the world of Canadian medicine, most doctors are self-employed, building a referral base for consultations and paying an office manager to take care of expenses. Doctors collect their fees from a single insurance company in each jurisdiction—the provincial or territorial government—and the fee for each consultation or procedure is strictly defined. The only way for a doctor to increase their income is to work more hours—or to become a specialist that delivers higher-cost procedures. Patients have no worries about insurance coverage, and doctors have no worries about getting paid. The patient's cost for visiting a doctor or using core hospital services is charged to the provincial government's medical insurance plan, which then pays the doctor or the hospital.

Doctors electronically submit claims to their provincial or territorial single-payer plan and are paid by direct deposit into their bank account. In contrast to medical practice in the United States, we don't employ collection agencies to chase unpaid medical bills.

Critics of Canada's system sometimes use the term "socialized medicine," but that is a misnomer. Unlike the UK's National Health Service (NHS), where physicians are employed by the government, most doctors in Canada, as I said, are self-employed. Canada's system is a mix of private providers billing governments for publicly funded services. Thus, it's better described as a "single-payer insurance system," given that doctors maintain a high degree of entrepreneurial freedom and professional autonomy.

Canada's health care system was born in Regina, Saskatchewan. Its introduction through a Saskatchewan Legislative Assembly Act triggered province-wide labour action in the summer of 1962 that lasted twenty-three days, with the striking doctors' supporters standing on the steps of the legislature threatening politicians. I remember this from my childhood, as well as the public panic that went along with it. Up to this point, doctors had always set their own fees and collected cash from their patients, and they didn't want to give that up. Eventually, Lord Taylor, a distinguished doctor-politician from England, was brought in as a mediator and brokered a deal to end the strike. Through a series of steps best explained by others,[1] a new system, unofficially called Medicare, was eventually adopted across Canada, and life went on.

Canadian Medicare today is much as it was in 1962. The provincial doctors' association—the Saskatchewan Medical Association—maintains a contract with the government and negotiates fees. For each unit of medical service—a ten-minute consultation, for example, or a

---

[1] Gregory P. Marchildon, ed., *Making Medicare: New Perspectives on the History of Medicare in Canada* (Toronto: University of Toronto Press, 2012).

surgical procedure—the physician collects a prescribed fee. A specialist in this system, even working part-time, makes enough to support office expenses and a comfortable lifestyle. Of course, some Canadian specialists—looking at their richest medical counterparts in the United States—would say it's not comfortable enough. But I will testify that some Saskatchewan doctors are in the top rank of local society, golf at expensive clubs, and enjoy fine holidays. They do not, to my knowledge, live north of the tracks among the patients, largely Indigenous people, who visit the Emergency units at Regina's hospitals, the Pasqua and the General.

Family doctors earn considerably less in this negotiated fee structure. This creates an incentive for them to maximize the number of patients they see to support their lifestyle. Fee-for-service medicine can become a treadmill with ten-minute visits back-to-back, though not all doctors practise this way. The treadmill is laborious and tiring, and many new graduates from medical schools in Canada are opting for a different pay structure. In 2023, the Ministry of Health in Saskatchewan announced implementation of a blended model for paying family physicians instead of the traditional fee-for-service model.[2] It is hoped that a different pay structure will allow physicians to spend more time with their patients.

---

2   Larissa Kurz, "Sask. Family Doctors Pleased with New Payment Model Proposal," *Regina Leader-Post*, May 9, 2023, https://leaderpost.com/health/sask-family-doctors-pleased-with-new-payment-model-proposal. The Ministry of Health announced a blended model, giving doctors a base payment for each patient on their roster, and if the patient needs more than the standard basket of services, the doctor will be paid an additional fee for the extra services. The model also calls for a redesign of the health care system in Saskatchewan with team-based care. As written by the presidents of the Saskatchewan Medical Association and the Saskatchewan College of Family Physicians, "Patients will receive the right care, at the right time, by the right member of the team." John Gjevre and Andries Muller, "Opinion: Physician-led, team-based care is path to better Sask. access," *Saskatoon StarPhoenix*, March 10, 2023, https://thestarphoenix.com/opinion/columnists/opinion-physician-led-team-based-care-is-path-to-better-sask-access.

Canada's health care system is better, in some ways, than the US system in which tens of millions of people are excluded from routine and non-emergency medical care except on a charity basis. This American system combines a hodge podge of government-funded programs for soldiers and their families, veterans, seniors (Medicare), the deserving poor (Medicaid), and elected politicians and their staff. But millions of Americans fall into the middle, unable to qualify for public assistance and unable to afford private insurance in the marketplace. This publicly funded patchwork of health care, together with a complex private pay insurance market, keeps hundreds of health insurance and health care companies profitable but creates a barrier between patients and their health care providers.

As of 2018, 34 percent of Americans received their health care through government programs.[3] Many Americans do not realize that their tax dollars, paid to federal and state governments, are covering a significant portion of health care. It is a partially socialized system, but Americans prickle at the word "socialism," so this fact is largely overlooked in public conversation.

Canada's publicly funded single-payer system has advantages. The overall cost of health care to the economy is far lower than in the US, but it still takes a significant bite from governments' budgets. All lawful residents of Canada have health coverage, including Treaty Indians, non-Treaty Indians, Métis, and Inuit. Nonetheless, Canada's system has many flaws. The demand for health care services is immense, especially if one considers scientific advances in the treatment of disease combined with an aging population. We have enough

---

3   Ryan Nunn, Jana Parsons, and Jay Shambaugh, "A Dozen Facts about the Economics of the US Health-Care System," Brookings Institution, March 10, 2020, https://www.brookings.edu/research/a-dozen-facts-about-the-economics-of-the-u-s-health-care-system/.

physicians per capita, in theory, but they tend to live in urban areas, and not in vast, low-density rural areas, and this creates a disparity in access. Most family physicians are tied to the fee-for-service model as independent small business owners, which requires them to own a practice, hire staff to run the office, and incentivizes them to see patients quickly to increase their compensation. The fee-for-service model can also result in physicians bringing in patients for easy, low-value visits during which they review issues that could be handled by phone, such as a routine result from a blood test. Family doctors often close their practices to new patients while foolishly insisting on doing tasks that could be done by others. This creates an apparent shortage of doctors, which is even more pronounced in Indigenous communities, where there may be only a nursing station or a visiting doctor once a month.

Surgical specialists, meanwhile, are limited by the availability of "operating room time," which describes a shortage of supporting staff, such as nurses. Appropriate allocation of resources is complex, and surgical wait-lists have become a political football in Canada.[4] More affluent patients may choose to fly to the United States or Mexico rather than wait for surgery in Canada, but the number of people doing this has been estimated to represent less than 0.1 percent of cases.[5]

The quality of care in our hospitals is excellent, whether surgical or otherwise, but the Canadian system is less effective in promoting good health at home, monitoring and responding to health issues in

---

4 Diana Duong, "How Can Canada Reduce Surgical Backlogs without Expanding Privatization?" *Canadian Medical Association Journal* 194, no. 44 (November 15, 2022), E1514–E1515, https://doi.org/10.1503/cmaj.1096025.
5 Steven J. Katz, Karen Cardiff, Marina Pascali, Morris L. Barer, and Robert G. Evans, "Phantoms in the Snow: Canadians' Use of Health Care Services in the United States," *Health Affairs* 21, no. 3 (May/June 2002), 19–31, https://doi.org/10.1377/hlthaff.21.3.19.

the community, and getting people to hospital on time.⁶ And for First Nations communities, the system has often been a failure.

When Saskatchewan set up its medical care insurance program in the 1960s, it was supposed to fit with the existing network of clinics and hospitals to provide health care coverage for every citizen, including Indigenous People. Unfortunately, there were no doctors' offices on Indigenous territories. Responsibility for Indigenous Peoples' health, going back to the founding of Canada in 1867, rests with the Government of Canada; but Canada shut down its shabby Indian hospitals before 1960 and has never really gotten around to providing a replacement. As described later in this book, health care clinics funded by the federal government on Indigenous reserves have grown up bit by bit, but medical doctors are not part of the package.

People living in the Indigenous territories often face a long list of barriers to maintaining good health and finding medical treatment. In most cases, their community lacks access to pharmacies, grocery stores, recreation, and decent housing. They may not have the means to travel to a doctor's office or an outpatient clinic. The result is that Indigenous health outcomes tend to be worse than those in non-Indigenous populations in almost every respect.

---

6 "[T]he Canadian healthcare system is designed around an acute care paradigm, where the focus is to address (rather than prevent) urgent issues and manage chronic illnesses. Acute illnesses tend to be short, diagnosed easily and treated with a cure. It makes perfect sense for this type of care to be provided reactively. Our system has excelled at providing—and needs to continue providing—reactive care in the context of acute illness…[However], this reactive approach to healthcare is both expensive and, to some degree, ineffective in meeting the needs of today's population, from the healthiest individual to the complex chronically ill." Alexis Wise, Emily MacIntosh, Nirusan Rajakulendran, and Zayna Khayat, "Transforming Health: Shifting from Reactive to Proactive and Predictive Care," MaRS Market Insights, March 29, 2016, https://www.marsdd.com/news/transforming-health-shifting-from-reactive-to-proactive-and-predictive-care/.

I returned to Saskatchewan to contribute to the community where I had grown up. I decided to put a large part of my effort into working at Regina General Hospital, which serves a combined urban and rural population from a wide geographic area. This is Saskatchewan's busiest hospital measured by the numbers of Emergency visits, admissions, and surgeries.[7]

The head of the Division of General Internal Medicine, Dr. Patrick Duffy, had put me on the call schedule a few days after my arrival. He arranged to meet me in the doctors' lounge. It was a Friday, and he threw me in at the deep end. I would be on call for the next seventy-two hours, working days and nights until Monday morning at 8:00 a.m. Arriving to begin my shift, I wore a white coat with a stethoscope and carried a pager and notepad in my pocket. My shiny new badge hung around my neck on a lanyard. Dr. Duffy was almost the same height as I am, at five feet eight inches; he was dressed in a button-down shirt and khaki pants, and sported a brush cut. His Irish accent and strong handshake were endearing and authoritative.

"So, when the ER calls you, you go to the ER and assess the patient," he told me. "I warn you our ER physicians make a lot of mistakes, so don't be fooled by them. Everyone that is admitted to the medical ward in the hospital is yours to take care of. Be sure to keep your yellow sheets so you can bill the consultation. You're responsible for all the admitted medical patients overnight on the wards, covering for our group of internists. We need the sleep because we've been worked to the bone. Be sure to yell at those nurses who call you for Tylenol in the middle of the night. Good luck!"

Despite twenty years of practising medicine and my confidence in my skills as a doctor, I was terrified that I would get lost in the hospital

---

7   Personal conversation with Dr. Gill White, associate dean of medicine, University of Saskatchewan.

connector hallways or make a wrong turn in my diagnostic thinking. I was the specialist in charge of internal medicine patients throughout a complex of more than four hundred beds, with only an uncertain amount of support from subspecialist colleagues, over a period of three days. When Patrick left, I remained behind in the doctors' lounge. I sat on the leather couch and stared at a painting of a cowboy on a horse in a summer prairie field, roping a calf to wrestle it to the ground. It was an action scene, a powerful image of the Western lifestyle. The equivalent painting in Eastern Canada would be one of the fall colours in Algonquin Park; or in British Columbia, the orcas playing in the Pacific Ocean. An hour later, rousing me from my thoughts of Canadian painting styles, my pager went off. I slid over to the phone on the side table next to the leather couch and called the number displayed on the pager. It was the ER.

The Emergency Room is the heart of any hospital. ER physicians triage patients, sending some home and deciding which of the others are sick enough to get into one of our precious hospital beds. When I arrived in the ER on this Friday night, the doc pulled me aside and said, "The guy in room five has a raging infection in his leg, blood cultures have been ordered, and I think he needs IV antibiotics." The need for intravenous antibiotics signals an automatic admission into hospital. I thanked my colleague and proceeded to room five.

My new patient, my first patient, was sitting on a gurney in a blue hospital gown with a sheet over his torso and legs. The chart said his name was Alvin. He was forty years old, lanky, with minimal facial hair, dark skin, and black hair. He had a toothless smile, and his hair was long and braided down to his mid-back. I introduced myself as the hospital's Internal Medicine specialist and asked, "Alvin, what brings you into the Emergency Room?"

He smiled weakly at me and said, "I was havin' problems walking."

"How long has this been going on?"

"'Bout two weeks, but it got worse over the last two days so I couldn't get out of bed. Then I started to see this redness streaking up my leg, and it really hurts, Doc." He pulled up the sheet covering his legs and showed me his right ankle, swollen, the size of a grapefruit, with blotches of red skin creeping up to mid-calf.

I examined him, asked him pertinent questions for the medical exam—previous history, previous surgeries, smoking, drinking—and explained that he would be admitted to the hospital for intravenous antibiotics. As I edged towards the door to leave the room, he said, "Hey, Doc, are you going to give me something for pain?" I turned to face him with a smile, but my inner reaction was one of suspicion. I was convinced that he was a drug-seeker, looking for an empathetic, naive physician to prescribe narcotics. I said, "Yes, I'll give you something for pain," knowing that I would order him Tylenol with no narcotics. He wasn't going to take me for a fool. I wasn't going to get drawn into being his enabler, I reasoned. As our relationship evolved over the next few days, I learned that I was wrong. So wrong. He was truly in pain, and as his infection improved, his desire for painkilling drugs subsided.

Sometime on Saturday morning, as I made a round through the medical ward, a doctor that I didn't recognize approached me to talk about Alvin's condition. He introduced himself as Dr. Stuart Skinner, a specialist in infectious diseases. He seemed quite young. In a gentle voice, he educated me: "I just checked his blood cultures in the lab. He's growing *Staph aureus*. He'll need intravenous antibiotics for two weeks. Have you checked his heart for infection on his heart valve? We have to put him in isolation; there's a risk that he could infect other patients in this ward." Since this was my first hospitalized patient in Regina, and I needed help to navigate the system, I appreciated his counsel. I thanked him for his advice—the normal response from a general internist to a subspecialist who can provide essential knowledge.

Isolation would put Alvin into a private room, a coveted perk that most patients request when coming to the hospital. When I saw him next, Alvin was settled comfortably with his own bathroom, an intravenous needle in his left arm for his daily antibiotic infusion. He appeared content. His eyes were deep and bright. He was receptive and warmed to seeing me. I checked his ankle and noticed that the swelling had decreased; what was once a grapefruit was now the size of a large orange. The red streaks were still present, but less vibrant.

Afterward, in the hallway outside his room, I ordered an echocardiogram to check for infection in his heart. I was greeted by the hospital's social worker, who let me know that Alvin was homeless, although he had a status card from a reserve near Regina. We both knew this reality to be a major contributor to any patient's health problems. Living on the streets is stressful; homeless people run a constant risk of violent assault, the loss of their few possessions and identification cards, and unsanitary conditions.

Homelessness is a circumstance associated with addictions, abuse, and poverty, often caused by or contributing to mental illness. In Saskatchewan, famously, the temperature may drop to below minus thirty degrees for days at a time. Even on this warm summer day, I would need the expertise of the social worker to help decide on a course of care.

I visited Alvin daily, and the infection slowly improved. His heart echo and blood cultures were negative, but he still needed intravenous antibiotics. On the fifth day, we had an eye-opening interaction. I re-asked the routine medical questions: How are you doing? (Fine.) Are you in pain? (No.) Are the antibiotics doing their job? (Yes.) Can you walk? (No, I need to use the wheelchair.) Our eyes glanced in unison to the wheelchair beside his bed. He looked at me and stated that he wanted to wander the hospital, but the nurses had confined him to his room. I glanced at his bedside table, and it was filled with books. I wondered aloud how he got them into his room, and he said a friend had brought them to him from the free bookshelf near the hospital lobby; he had finished them, and he needed more.

We approach all relationships with a collection of images from our past. The books at Alvin's bedside brought back a childhood memory of visiting the Regina Public Library. Every Saturday, from the age of ten until I entered high school, my girlfriend and I would walk two blocks to a city bus stop and ride north. The twenty-five-minute trip took us from quiet crescents, with comfortable houses set well back from the street, into a downtown grid of office buildings and retail stores. The new library seemed vast, a modern structure with steel struts and walls of glass. We would carefully select four library books—that was the limit—and then proceed to the nearby Novia Café, facing Victoria Park, where we enjoyed a feast of chips and gravy. My free time throughout the next week would be spent reading the books I had discovered. For me, those books brought the excitement of travel—on a childish scale—combined with the warmth and safety of escaping into fiction.

I looked more closely at the books on Alvin's table: Ernest Hemingway, F. Scott Fitzgerald, John Steinbeck. Sophisticated titles, classic twentieth-century fare—they took me by surprise. I glanced from the books to his face. "These are interesting books. How did you develop your taste in reading?" Internally, I was checking my view of First Nations people as uneducated and simple, hoping my question would not offend him.

"I grew up in Hollywood and went to a school in LA," he stated simply. Caught off guard by this statement, I was able to contain my surprise. Many years ago, I had visited LA with my ex-husband, and I didn't recall having noticed any Indigenous people on the street. I returned my focus to Alvin; I realized that I was his doctor and didn't need this information to solve his medical situation—we had now slipped into social conversation. And I had other patients to see.

Due to hospital rules, written and enforced by the Infection Control office, I couldn't allow Alvin out of his room. But I did stop by the free bookshelf and brought more books to his room every time I visited.

After two weeks, Alvin's infection was resolved. The hospital social worker found him a room in temporary housing in the city. I wish I could report that Alvin reconnected with his extended family and entered a process of stability, but I don't know that. Our relationship ended at the hospital's front door.

This brief interaction with Alvin, coming so soon after my return to Saskatchewan, pushed me to examine my attitudes. I realized that despite my abstract desire to help and support Indigenous people, I had been painting them all with the same brush. I had been making assumptions about a common personality type and a common backstory. I realized that I needed to learn more about how the fragmentation of Indigenous society had affected individual people. I began to explore the story of colonialism from first contact, and the effects of colonialism on Indigenous Peoples that resonate still today.

A FIELD ON THE PRAIRIE

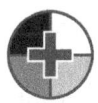

The elevator door opens, and I walk out into a long corridor. I'm still feeling that this hospital is new to me. I'm not settled in. My thoughts are scattered. I'm focused on getting home after work and making an overdue phone call to a friend in Lancaster, Pennsylvania, three thousand kilometres away.

Ahead of me I hear the voice of a woman, agitated, shouting in Cree.

Outside, it is a bright, cold, windy fall day. The city rolls away from the hospital in every direction, the legislature and the most affluent streets in the south and east, the railway tracks and the poorest districts to the north. Surrounding it all is the south Saskatchewan plain: flat, almost treeless, drawn into neat grids of roads, fences, and cultivated farms. Harvest is in full swing and the crops are golden. Inside, everything is beige or stark white with fluorescent light. Neutral. Antiseptic. Institutional.

I enter the room where my patient waits. She is sitting up in bed, picking at something in the air, dark eyes blazing. Her husband and middle-aged son are sitting on institutional chairs close by, wearing tired, forlorn faces. The patient calms somewhat when I enter the room in my uniform—the white lab coat, the stethoscope. "Mavis, do you remember meeting me last night?" I ask. Her eyes harden, and I see a serpent eating at her soul. "You are the devil," she says. The previous evening, she was coherent but far away, telling me in clipped English that she was crossing a field on the prairie, walking with her father, watching the buffalo. Now she has grown intense, and she is angry with me.

Mavis arrived from her reserve in the Touchwood Hills late on the previous day, a frail woman in her mid-seventies bundled into an ambulance, driven for two hours, and deposited in the Emergency Room with a dangerously elevated INR at 28.[1] A normal INR level is 1, or between 2 and 3 for patients on anticoagulants; a level as high as 28 is often associated with death from internal bleeding. A CT scan of her head, performed after she was admitted, showed no obvious bleeding in her brain to explain the confusion. I ordered reversal agents to thicken the blood, and this morning her INR indicated normal clotting. We have fixed the cause of her abnormal blood tests, but she is not better. She is now my patient, and I need to consider how her anger might be related to her medical symptoms. She has heart disease with atrial fibrillation. Thinning the blood to prevent a stroke was what I judged to be the appropriate treatment for her heart disease, but it may be that the treatment has become life-threatening. In order to heal her, I have to understand why her blood was so thinned in the first place. Was it alcohol use, kidney failure, confusion about dosing, a suicide attempt?

I turn away from Mavis as she fends off the serpent inside her, and I focus on the family at her bedside. Her husband is a heavy-set man wearing a beaded jacket and blue jeans, his long greyish hair in a braid

---

[1] INR is the international normalized ratio that measures the effect of anticoagulants on the clotting system. It is usually used to measure the effect of warfarin, an oral anticoagulant, on the thinness of the blood.

down his back. He tells me he is an Elder on the reserve and does pipe ceremonies. They have been married for many years. He says she has been taking her heart pills regularly, but there is no evidence she intentionally took too many. *Checkmark: strike suicide attempt off the list.* She is not a drinker. *Checkmark: strike alcohol interaction with her pills off the list.* From a review of her blood work in the hospital chart, I can see her kidneys are working well. *Checkmark: strike kidney failure off the list.*

Still, she is sick, and she is angry. I suspect that she has every reason to be angry, aside from her illness, although I have never experienced racism or real deprivation myself. I grew up in a comfortable home, surrounded at school by white faces, steeped in a culture that celebrated the bravery and enterprise of the early settlers—the men and women who broke the soil, the doctors and police officers. As I passed through college in the early 1970s, a truer perspective started to emerge. I learned about the Canadian government's treaties with Indigenous Peoples in Saskatchewan.

Shortly after the time of Canadian Confederation, the Hudson's Bay Company transferred the governance of Rupert's Land to the government of Canada, under pressure from Great Britain, for a price. Through two centuries of fur trading, the Hudson's Bay Company had transformed the pattern of economic activity among Indigenous people, but the land stretching from the Pacific coast through much of what is currently Ontario still lay open for traditional use. There were no police or government agents in the early fur trading days. On July 1, 1867, the British North America Act created the Dominion of Canada, a self-governing entity within the British Empire. Suddenly, the Crown appeared, in the form of an Ontario-based Conservative government, intent on transforming the prairies into a replica of southern Ontario. The treaties, along with the Indian Act, were the government's key instruments in clearing the land for settlement. Through Treaty 4, the Canadians seized the field where Mavis, in her visions, watched buffalo.

They carved up the prairie landscape and put Mavis's people on reserves. Treaty 4 was signed by her ancestors at Fort Qu'Appelle in 1874—two years before Custer's Last Stand, the Battle of the Little Bighorn, in what is now the state of Montana. Over a century later, the Truth and Reconciliation Commission called this process of treaty-making part of Canada's "cultural genocide."[2]

It is an indication of the strength and resilience of Indigenous people like Mavis that they have survived and often showed a talent for succeeding in the world that was forced upon them by the settlers intent on westward expansion. Saskatchewan's Poundmaker Reserve was the birthplace of Hollywood star Gordon Tootoosis; the Red Pheasant Reserve was home to the accomplished Indigenous artist Allen Sapp; and Maria Campbell, who became a lifelong advocate for Indigenous arts and politics, was born on a trap line in northwestern Saskatchewan.

The Chief from Mavis's homeland in the Touchwood Hills was party to signing Treaty 4 in 1874. He remained Chief of his band until his death nearly twenty years later.

When the treaty was signed, the Chief and his council carefully chose heavily wooded land to give them access to wild game and firewood in the harsh prairie environment. Cultivation was done at that time using spades and hoes; a plot known as the "community garden" was maintained by the whole reserve. The community developed a fine herd of cattle, each farmer keeping his herd until it numbered ten to twelve heads, and then giving half of the animals to someone else who could then get started. After the band received walking ploughs, its members began to grow wheat, barley, and oats; with the arrival of the railway in

---

[2] Truth and Reconciliation Commission of Canada, "Honouring the Truth, Reconciling for the Future: Summary of the final report of the Truth and Reconciliation Commission of Canada," Truth and Reconciliation Commission of Canada, 2015, 1. The full report can be accessed online at https://publications.gc.ca/collections/collection_2015/trc/IR4-7-2015-eng.pdf.

the early 1900s, an outlet was created for the sale of their produce. In the 1940s, the band purchased their first tractor.

They worked hard on a cramped piece of land that was less than ideal for farming, and they persevered. The "white chiefs" had promised a "medicine chest" in Treaty 6 signed at Fort Carlton in 1876, but the federal government's health care efforts in the first half of the twentieth century were less than minimal. Indigenous children were taken, some at gunpoint, to live in residential schools where they risked death from tuberculosis, other infectious diseases, starvation, and abuse. Housing on reserve was provided rarely and unpredictably, with no resources for maintenance.

Using my medical skills and training, I conclude that Mavis is suffering from white matter disease and explain my findings to her husband. The brain has several parts—the grey matter is where cognitive functions happen, and the white matter is the connective fibres that link the various parts of the brain, just as a railroad track connects two cities. Mavis's CT scan indicates that she has evidence of small vessel disease in the brain that is associated with dementia, balance problems, and difficulty with multitasking. It worsens with infection or stress. It is likely that as her mild dementia tipped over into severe dementia, she was unaware of the progressive decline and mistakenly took too many of her pills, which would explain why her blood was so thinned. There is no treatment for white matter disease, except to improve the underlying stressful situation. With rest, good nutrition, controlling blood pressure, and exercise, the symptoms improve with time. Her husband accepts my explanation but does not seem convinced that she will improve.

Over the next short while I return to Mavis's room daily. Her husband sits by her bedside for three days. She grows stronger and interacts with the staff and me. Her son is also visiting. Her daughter flies into Regina from her job in Toronto.

On the fourth day she is alone. She smiles at me, is well groomed and sitting comfortably in bed. Her blood work has normalized, and she is calm in her speech. Her caring family has disappeared. And she is alone.

Where have they gone? I begin to suspect a case of "granny dumping." This term was coined in the 1980s by medical professionals who observed relatives dropping off the elderly in Emergency Rooms when the family was unable or unwilling to care for them due to burnout or lack of financial resources. Granny dumping typically peaks before long weekends or at Christmas. It is spoken of as a widespread condition in the health care system; it creates a dilemma for physicians and social workers reluctant to discharge a patient when a family is absent or doesn't show up for meetings with the hospital staff. I become convinced that this pleasant family has hoodwinked me. I had mistakenly thought they cared for Mavis. I feel irritation with myself at my blind trust.

Four days later, Mavis's husband reappears. I find him sitting calmly by her bedside. I hide my irritation over his apparent abandonment and respond to him carefully and professionally. I explain that she has improved further and will soon be ready to go home. We are waiting for one last test on her heart. She will likely be discharged tomorrow. I ask her husband, "Are you okay with that?"

He smiles gracefully with this news. Then he looks me in the eye and says, "I'm sorry that I couldn't be here for the last few days. We had a crisis on reserve. One of our young girls was found in a ditch after being raped and killed. We had religious services to honour her."

I am embarrassed and ashamed. I had been caught up in my privileged view of appropriate behaviour while the community on reserve was grieving the loss of one of its youth and reeling in the face of the violence against her. He tells me that the culprits were likely non-Indigenous, the details are fuzzy, and no one has been caught yet. I had fallen into the trap of making assumptions about Indigenous people and granny dumping. I am on a path of discovering my own racism.

+ + +

I am reminded as I write this of a study on the Vitals website that reported on the results of interviews with the public to determine what makes a good physician.[3] Patients listed the following characteristics: confidence, empathy, a humane approach, personal interest, respect, and thoroughness. I like to think that I possess all these qualities, but there are some key ingredients missing from the survey. First, it strangely ignores the technical competence that allowed me to diagnose Mavis's condition. Second, and more important for this account, is the question of cultural barriers—such as my own ignorance of the realities of Indigenous life—and their effects on the quality of medical care.

Within a few weeks of meeting Mavis and her family, I made the decision to remain in Regina and work at the Regina General Hospital, recognizing that it was built on Treaty 4 territory without permission from the original caretakers of the land. After years away from home, I had embarked on a reconciliation journey.

In a way, it had started ten years earlier while I was assistant professor of medicine at Duke University in Durham, North Carolina. The message to return to Saskatchewan came out of the blue and from an expected source: a professional career counsellor. While re-evaluating my career goals, my boss suggested that I consult the Center for Professional Wellbeing at an office nearby the university. I realized that I had nothing to lose by meeting the director at the centre, Dr. Pfifferling. On a sunny, humid afternoon, he asked me about my background, my family, my work situation, and my dreams. I told him that I came from

---

3   Vitals is a subdivision of the WebMD website, hosted by dedicated experts in the field, that matches patients with physicians; one of their surveys polled 2,319 adults about their personalities, rapport with current doctors, and preferences in a health care provider. https://www.vitals.com.

a small city in Western Canada; my medical degree, although valid, is from a medical school not widely known in the US. I told him about my personal struggle with finances, with the prolonged legal battle over custody. I confessed to him about the imposter syndrome that I was experiencing at one of the most prestigious universities in the States. I told him about my dreams of doing something significant with my life. I spoke about ambition, persistence, and curiosity about the world. He listened carefully and thoughtfully. He was a renowned speaker and had just come back from a conference in Canada where he had met an Indigenous spiritual advisor. His advice to me was unexpected: go back to Canada and work in Indigenous health care, he said. I walked out of his office, a little shaken from his advice to take such a left-hand turn. I had grants to be funded, academic papers to finish, and students to teach. I put his advice aside.

It took me years to realize he was right. In 2011 I packed up my winter clothes, computer, and medical degrees; I found a tenant for my house in Lancaster, Pennsylvania. After decades in academic medicine, I began work as a community physician in the city where I had started my career as an idealistic medical student.

My interactions with Indigenous people in the Saskatchewan health care system have made me examine my beliefs and my behaviour. I am not alone in this journey. When I attend conferences, academic events, or public gatherings, it has become customary to begin with a land acknowledgement, which recognizes the traditional territory of the Indigenous Peoples from whom we settlers have taken so much. It's a start, but we must do much more than pay respects.

A MIDDLE GROUND

Kathleen is a beautiful nineteen-year-old—olive skin, dark hair swept up in a chignon-like bun that accentuates her soft yet sharp cheekbones. She has arrived at my outpatient office on Albert Street for an appointment. Her dark eyes sparkle when she talks. I am sitting behind my desk, white coat on, stethoscope around my neck. She is sitting facing the desk with legs crossed. Flowing skirt, low cut top with high cleavage. There is a tattoo peeping through her loose blouse at her left shoulder. As I strain to see the tattoo, I notice a small, almost imperceptible swelling on the left side of her neck; it appears to be an injection point for intravenous drugs.

I ask her if she has plans for her future. Softly and with some shyness she says, "I want to be a doctor."

I say, "I hope that can happen for you." I ask her to come to the exam table so we can finish our medical exam.

I met Kathleen at the ER a week earlier when I was on call. She had come to the hospital with chest pain, but no heart disease was found. Instead she had a skin infection, often called cellulitis, requiring intravenous antibiotics. This is a follow-up visit to check on her infection.

My office is at the edge of the downtown core, on a bus route, in a space shared with five other doctors, and it runs at full tilt. We have cramped examination rooms, tight hallways, and a small waiting room always overflowing with patients. When I'm not in the ER or elsewhere in the hospital, I am at the office.

I am qualified as a general internist. An American College of Physicians logo says, perhaps unhelpfully: *Internists—Doctors for Adults*. Most people don't know what a general internist does. I sometimes explain: heart, lungs, kidneys, all the internal organs. Most of the time, they don't care. They just want someone competent to care for their illness. They don't want to know about my post-doctoral studies or extra training. I have the expertise to manage the very sick, but in my work in the hospital ER, which spills over to the Albert Street practice, I see patients at all levels of illness or injury.

Kathleen has walked here through the streets of the inner city. It is late August and is a "Three Bears" day: not too hot, not too cold, just right. She climbs up on the exam table, and I have an opportunity to examine her neck. As I suspected, the small punctate scar in her neck vein shows that she has injected drugs. She has a heart murmur. She tells me how much better she feels after receiving antibiotics. She denies any fevers or chills. The leg cellulitis she had in the hospital is resolved. The infection has cleared. We finish the exam, and she leaves. The next time I see her, the dream of becoming a doctor will seem much further away.

What is Kathleen's background? She moved to the city with her mother, two young brothers, and a young sister when she was twelve years old, from one of the dozens of Indigenous Nations scattered along the dirt roads of southern Saskatchewan. She survived her teenage years in the city under the protection of her mother and aunties, landing jobs serving coffee and fast food until she passed the age of sixteen. Along the way, she developed a fashion sense borrowed from her friends and from magazines and movies. When I met her she was struggling, but I thought her underlying health was strong, and I hoped—based on my growing but still limited understanding of the barriers facing Indigenous people—for the best for her.

+ + +

Family lore holds that I am a descendant of Titameg, a Swampy Cree woman from the area around York Factory on James Bay. I learned this when I was in my teens, after a cousin decided to research our family tree.

Titameg married John Favel, who worked as a factor at the Hudson Bay Company's Fort Albany between 1740 and 1784. One of their daughters, Mary, married trader John McKay in 1791. They moved to Brandon House, a Hudson's Bay trading post on the prairie far to the south; Titameg, the matriarch, also settled there after her husband's death. After a couple of generations, another Mary McKay (1852–1928) married another fur trader, Alexander Campbell (1844–1925), born in Stornoway on the Isle of Lewis, Scotland. He left the fur trade and took up farming during the first wave of European settlement in the Saskatchewan parkland, choosing land near Prince Albert on the North Saskatchewan River. Their youngest son, Colin, was my grandfather. Through DNA testing, my mother learned that she was about 10 percent Indigenous.

I remember talking this over with my mother in the late 1960s. I remember feeling proud that we could claim "Indian" blood, but even as a young child I recognized that shame had also infiltrated our family. My mother told me the story in a low voice, an indicator to a small child that it was a secret. I watched her with other adults, and she never mentioned it to them. It was like a stain that needed to be hidden. My father, on the other hand, used to loudly talk about his "life with the Indians" followed by a barrel laugh that filled the house. Whenever my father made this statement, my mother would roll her eyes. She often laughed at his other jokes, but not this one.

In reflecting on this family history many years later, I took the time to read some written accounts of the relationships among First Nations, fur traders, and their Métis descendants. From the start of the organized fur trade in the 1670s, most fur traders came from Scotland or Quebec. The Scots might travel back to their homeland, and some Indigenous wives lived out their lives in Scotland. More often, the fur trader worked at different posts during his career, taking his Indigenous wife along with him. One defining feature of this history appears to be the adoption of "white ways" by the Indigenous women and a loss of cultural identification with their Indigenous background. I believe this is what happened in my family. Indians were believed to be lazy and heathenish in the European-dominated culture of British North America; hiding her origins would enable an improvement in status for an Indigenous woman.

Late on a Wednesday afternoon in February 2016, I learned that Senator Murray Sinclair was delivering the annual Woodrow Lloyd Lecture at the University of Regina. Sinclair had been raised by his grandparents on a reserve; eventually he was called to the bar and rose to the Manitoba Court of Queen's Bench. Over a period of six years, he had chaired Canada's Truth and Reconciliation Commission, and the final report had just been released. I donned my winter coat and boots and walked from my house to the Education Auditorium, arriving about five minutes before the lecture was to begin. The hall was full, with reserved rows at the front for Indigenous dignitaries, and only odd seats available. Luckily, I was solo and able to find a place, rather than be relegated to the overflow room to watch on video.

The lecture started with a prayer and smudge, blessing the land we were on, and recognizing the Treaty 4 nations as well as the Survivors of the residential schools. When Justice Sinclair spoke, he commanded attention with a folksy, personal style. He interwove his story with descriptions of the hard work that was done to produce the Truth and Reconciliation report. I was struck by his statement that he grew up "white," becoming valedictorian for his high school class, and, with ambition, achieved career success.

Murray Sinclair knew he was Indigenous—he did not need to be told by a cousin—but growing up in Manitoba in the 1950s and '60s, he learned the shame associated with his cultural heritage. In his lecture, he talked about growing up with his grandmother. She would not allow him to speak their native language at home. When he asked why, he was told it was so he could be saved. Since the Catholic Church had taught that Indigenous traits were heathen, the only hope that Sinclair's grandmother had for her offspring was to deny them their Aboriginal roots. She wanted her offspring to go to heaven, of course.

The commission's *Final Report of the Truth and Reconciliation Commission of Canada*, issued in 2015, shone a spotlight on the atrocities that marked the attempted cultural genocide at the centre of the settler project in Canada. The residential schools, a key strategy in the attempted genocide, brought trauma that persists to this day. On the settler side, the existence of the residential schools was ignored for decades. In school, we studied the Confederation Poets, men such as Duncan Campbell Scott who promoted a new vision of Canada in the late 1800s ("Once in the winter / Out on a lake /...A Chippewa woman / With her sick baby / Crouched in the last hours / Of a great storm / Frozen and hungry..."). We did not learn that Scott was a senior federal government official who helped to introduce the residential school system and who campaigned explicitly for the extermination of Indigenous languages and cultures.

There is rising recognition of the crimes of Canada's past, but the question of how our health care system should address the resulting trauma is far from resolved. National surveys from Statistics Canada show that the overall health of the Indigenous population is significantly worse than that of the non-Indigenous population.[1] First Nations have double the infant mortality rate compared to the non-Aboriginal population.[2] The suicide rate for Indigenous youth is eleven times the national average. Adults have double the smoking rate and higher levels of asthma and chronic obstructive lung disease. Children are exposed to second-hand smoke and have higher rates of asthma. The obesity rate for Indigenous people is 26 percent, compared to 16 percent in the non-Indigenous population. The rate of diabetes is five times the national average, with women and people on reserve more affected.[3] There is a tremendous burden of infectious disease, with rising rates of tuberculosis (TB), Hepatitis C, and human immunodeficiency virus (HIV).

Perhaps there is room in Canadian society and in health care to find a middle ground—a place where exchange will happen between two cultures, a place of successful hybridization where "neither group has the ability to dominate the other."[4] The process could be one of mediation and understanding the roles of atonement, gift giving, and trade. Richard White's book about the Iroquois and fur traders provides a classic description of how Indigenous people and incomers sometimes found common meaning in the years before the establishment of the Canadian state:

---

[1] Chantelle A.M. Richmond and Catherine Cook, "Creating Conditions for Canadian Aboriginal Health Equity: The Promise of Healthy Public Policy," *Public Health Review* 37, no. 2 (July 20, 2016), https://doi.org/10.1186/s40985-016-0016-5.

[2] Z. Luo, R. Wilkins, J. Smylie, P. Martens, and W. Fraser, "Community Report: Community Characteristics and Birth Outcomes among First Nations and Non-First Nations in Manitoba, 1991–2000," 2007.

[3] Y. Mao, B.W. Moloughney, R.M. Semenciw, and H.I. Morrison, "Indian Reserve and Registered Indian Mortality in Canada," *Canadian Journal of Public Health* 83, no. 5 (September–October 1992), 350–353, https://pubmed.ncbi.nlm.nih.gov/1473061/.

[4] Richard White, *The Middle Ground: Indians, Empires, and Republics in the Great Lakes Region, 1650–1815* (New York: Cambridge University Press, 2011).

Diverse peoples adjust their differences through what amounts to a process of creative, and often expedient, misunderstandings. People try to persuade others who are different from themselves by appealing to what they perceive to be the values and practices of those others. They often misinterpret and distort both the values and the practices of those they deal with, but from these misunderstandings arise new meanings and through them new practices—the shared meanings and practices of the middle ground.⁵

Two weeks after our meeting in my office, Kathleen is back in hospital, occupying a bed in the ER. As a teacher in the College of Medicine, I spend part of my week instructing medical students, interns, and residents during their Internal Medicine rotation in the hospital. It is a big team this evening, with a senior resident, a junior resident, a family practice resident, and four medical students. We are collectively taking an overnight shift, on call for any Internal Medicine patients who may need admission to the hospital. The big board in the ER is lit up with names of patients already in rooms. The waiting room is full.

I assign a fourth-year medical student, Sarah, to examine Kathleen while I visit other ER patients with the rest of the team. A lady with a stroke, a man with difficulty breathing, a man with swollen legs. An hour later, I meet up with Sarah, a tall blonde wearing scrubs and a short white coat, at the desk at the hub of the ER. She presents the case to me before we enter Kathleen's room: "This is a twenty-year-old Aboriginal female who came to ER complaining of chest pain. She has

---

5   White, xxvi.

an enlarged spleen and bruising on physical exam. The labs show anemia, neutropenia, and thrombocytopenia."

I ask Sarah to formulate a differential diagnosis. "What are the possible causes of chest pain?"

She responds by reciting a list: "This patient could have pneumonia, pulmonary embolism, or heart attack."

"So what do you think is causing the abnormal lab results and bruising?" I ask.

"Leukemia," she answers. I am stone-faced, no expression. I don't want to let the student know what I am thinking. I know that her learning experience will be heightened by her own integration of physical findings, rather than having me tell her the answer. I don't know the right answer, but I do know that leukemia is unlikely. In fact, it is so unlikely that I am embarrassed for the student.

With Sarah in tow, I walk into the exam room to check her findings. Kathleen smiles brightly at me, remembering me from previous visits, but she looks pale and in distress. I ask her: "What happened?" She states that she is having chest pain, that it hurts when she breathes. There is the scent of alcohol on her breath as she speaks. I gently lift her hospital gown to examine her. Her chest is black and blue. I look her in the eye: "Did someone beat you up?" She turns her head towards the stark-white wall in the small examination room and whispers, "Yes, my boyfriend beat me up." Still facing that wall, she begins to cry.

I realize the weight of the factors that overwhelm her and prevent her from escaping her present situation—poor parenting by residential school Survivors, struggles with housing, inadequate schooling, few successful role models, inner pain soothed by alcohol and drugs, and a need for love. She has natural beauty and a sweet personality. She is lovable. She needs to leave her boyfriend, but between her social circle of urban friends and her family, she will find it difficult to escape the trap of abuse. She could go to a homeless shelter, but without money and a job, her prospects of surviving are dismal. Kathleen is struggling to survive in a world where there is limited support for her, either from social service agencies or from an Indigenous family that is no longer in the picture.

These thoughts run through my mind as I hold her hand. But right now I must focus on the medical aspects of her situation and leave the social determinants of her situation to later—even though the situation is having a profound effect on me. I feel ineffective. I do not have the tools to help her. I cannot effect the changes required to make her life better. All I can do is apply a bandage and send her home.

Sarah stands nearby, silent. She has completely missed the significance of the black and blue marks on Kathleen's chest and applied a strictly medical model. And yes, it was just possible that an underlying leukemia could have produced blood abnormalities that resulted in the bruising, although it was more likely related to alcohol abuse; the underlying social factors of the bruises were not considered. I step back into the teaching mode in a Socratic style—the student has observed my interaction with Kathleen. Sarah has likely had all the advantages offered by the white settler community: loving supportive parents, good public education, stable homelife, easy acceptance to university, a reasonably secure future as a doctor—very little to none of which applies to the patient. But Sarah's eyes have been opened to Kathleen's situation, and she has moved to a middle ground—where observation and empathy are as valuable as book learning in medicine.

TWO-EYED SEEING

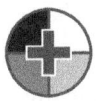

Soon after I returned to Regina to practise medicine, I received a seven-page handwritten complaint from a patient's family.

For several days, this kept me awake when I went home at night; in Canada's health care system, receiving a patient complaint is the equivalent of getting sued in the United States. It affects your reputation because it is reported to your department head. It may have implications for your medical licence. Beyond that, it calls into question the care you have delivered. It hurts emotionally. It bruises the ego. Some of my colleagues apparently have thicker skin than I do; I've learned over time that others receive many patient complaints. This fact doesn't console me.

The complaint, sent to the hospital's client representative, came from an Indigenous mother—let's call her Mrs. D—whose twenty-eight-year-old daughter died while under my care. In her letter, the mother expressed anger towards me and our health system. It named me, the medical students, and the nurses who worked on the case; we were, in her opinion, uncompassionate, inhumane, and had been unresponsive to her daughter's needs.

I felt empathy for that mother who had lost a daughter—along with fear and concern for myself, and a measure of surprise. The young woman had come to us with heart failure after living a turbulent life. She was a person who used drugs and alcohol. We applied for a heart transplant, but the surgeon turned her down because of her past non-compliance with medical treatments. After several meetings, her family appeared to understand that her heart failure was not treatable; she died peacefully with them at her bedside.

Soon after this, Mrs. D wrote a letter that accused me of treating her daughter as if she were a specimen, an object of medical experimentation. There were many physicians involved in her daughter's care, but I was the focus of her anger. Hospital management directed me to write a "Patient Service Recovery Letter" to pacify Mrs. D and diffuse her anger. They provided a checklist to follow: personalize the letter, thank the complainant for sharing their concerns, respond to the concerns in a factual, respectful, and honest manner, and apologize.

I struggled. What could I say, other than that I was sorry? Was it our fault that the young woman had skipped her medications and continued to abuse alcohol, despite our warnings? And yet I recognized that someone from a more privileged neighbourhood may have lived longer. I pointed this out to the cardiologist on the case, and he nodded. The mother's complaint made me think harder about my interactions with Indigenous people.

It's difficult to care for patients when they don't take care of themselves. As a physician, it makes me feel powerless. However, studies have shown that the patient's experience is often much worse. The patient who undergoes testing and probing and questioning from multiple physicians often feels like they are receiving less communication and care, not more. And if they react with frustration, many physicians push them away.

The medicine chest clause—the clause in Canada's Treaty 6 (1876) inserted by the lieutenant-governor of the territories, Commissioner

Alexander Morris—promised health care to Indigenous people. In a display of their ignorance of the differences between Indigenous Peoples of the region—a lack of understanding that Indigenous people often struggle against to this day—the commissioners who negotiated the treaties regarded the western plains groups such as the Anishinaabe, Cree, Saulteaux, and Assiniboine as one large entity, since they were intermarried and allied. Thanks to activism and legal action by Indigenous people in recent times, the federal government has moved, although slowly, towards fulfilling their promise; Métis people and Inuit are also covered by the programs created since 1960. Suspicion and resentment, however, persist. Indigenous people in the nineteenth century suffered and died from smallpox, tuberculosis, and starvation.[1] The historical narrative continues to hold the white man responsible for these diseases.

Through the first two-thirds of the twentieth century, a racist federal government treated Indigenous people as wards of the state. The Department of Indian Affairs established racially segregated Indian hospitals; the last such hospital was desegregated only in 1981. At these hospitals, patients were separated from their families and cared for by staff who had no training in Indigenous culture. There are reports of abuse, similar to the abuse reported in residential schools.

Canada's hospitals are now integrated, but Indigenous people still face poor outcomes when compared with others. The news stories and social media accounts are everywhere—snide remarks by hospital staff, delays in treatment, poor communication by physicians, unnecessary death. In 2017, media outlets called the story of Brian Sinclair—an Indigenous man who sat in a Winnipeg waiting room for thirty-four hours without being seen—a case of being "ignored to death."[2] My

---

[1] James W. Daschuk, *Clearing the Plains: Disease, Politics of Starvation, and the Loss of Aboriginal Life* (Regina: University of Regina Press, 2013).
[2] Aidan Geary, "Ignored to Death: Brian Sinclair's Death Caused by Racism,...

Indigenous patients know, even if they don't say it, that too many Indigenous patients leave hospital in a casket.

These issues are linked to the scarcity of health care in rural and remote areas. A Saskatchewan Conservative government moved to shore up its rural vote in the 1980s with the construction of sophisticated community hospitals in small towns, and this, along with other financial blunders, drove the province deep into debt. Consequently, many of these hospitals were closed by a New Democratic Party (NDP) government in the 1990s, and in my opinion, the NDP is still paying the price for that decision, unable to win a single rural legislative seat. Despite the lack of services in rural Saskatchewan, the governing Conservatives have not reopened the small-town hospitals. A sensible alternative would be to provide affordable transportation to the city for people in rural areas. For many years Saskatchewan had a unique province-wide bus system, funded and operated by the government, but the Saskatchewan Party (Conservatives under a new brand) eliminated funding for Saskatchewan Transportation in 2017, loading costs onto the sick and making access to medical care even more difficult. Although the rural residents are upset about this, a viable alternative government has not been elected in Saskatchewan.

With long wait times for specialist appointments and non-urgent elective surgeries in hospital, and with transportation barriers, people in Saskatchewan's villages, reserves, and remote northern communities are underserved. Given the lack of public transportation, the best approach—for now—is for health care professionals to take their expertise to the people who need it. A big part of this effort must be focused on helping individuals and communities to become more self-reliant.

...Inquest Inadequate, Group Says," CBC News, September 18, 2017, https://www.cbc.ca/news/canada/manitoba/winnipeg-brian-sinclair-report-1.4295996.

As I looked into the relationship between the medical system and Turtle Island's Indigenous people, I came across the concept of the Medicine Wheel.[3] Some authorities credit this phrase to non-Indigenous North Americans; Chief Robert Joseph says the term used by his people was *Sacred Circle*.[4] Whatever its origins, the term has been embraced by academics in the Indigenous Studies movement to promote understanding around health and healing.[5]

The Medicine Wheel embodies the four directions of the compass, as well as Father Sky, Mother Earth, and Spirit Tree—all symbolizing aspects of health and the cycles of life. Movement in the Medicine Wheel is circular, in a clockwise, or "sun-wise," direction. This aligns the human quest for health with the forces of nature, such as gravity and the rising and setting of the sun. Often the Medicine Wheel is described as physical, emotional, mental, and spiritual. The circle shape represents the interconnectivity of all parts of the human condition and their relationship with the elements of nature.

The wheel symbol figures in many of the traditions of the plains First Nations communities, as I learned when I attended my first powwow.

---

3   Lewis Mehl-Madrona, MD, of Cherokee-European descent, is a widely published medical doctor and researcher who has made a practice of combining Western medical treatments with holistic and Indigenous methods of treatment. Native American healing practices are described in his books *Coyote Medicine* (New York: Scribner, 1997) and *Coyote Wisdom: The Power of Story in Healing* (Rochester, VT: Bear & Co., 2005).

4   Chief Robert Joseph, "What Is an Indigenous Medicine Wheel," Indigenous Corporate Training Inc., May 24, 2020, www.ictinc.ca/blog/what-is-an-indigenous-medicine-wheel.

5   Angela Mashford-Pringle and Amy Shawanda, "Using the Medicine Wheel as Theory, Conceptual Framework, Analysis, and Evaluation Tool in Health Research," *SSM—Qualitative Research in Health* 3 (June 2023), 100251, https://doi.org/10.1016/j.ssmqr.2023.100251; Annie Wenger-Nabigon, "The Cree Medicine Wheel as an Organizing Paradigm of Theories of Human Development," *Native Social Work Journal* 7 (2010), 139–161, https://www.collectionscanada.gc.ca/obj/thesescanada/vol2/OSUL/TC-OSUL-387.pdf.

This event happened more than three years after I received the letter from Mrs. D, at the George Gordon First Nation community in the Touchwood Hills in Treaty 4 territory. Two colleagues and I drove from Regina and parked in a hayfield alongside a baseball stadium with wooden spectator stands. We could see from the licence plates on the cars parked around the baseball field that people had arrived from various jurisdictions across the Canadian prairies, the northern United States, and beyond.

We met our hosts behind the stands. Twenty or thirty men and women were waiting beside them in full regalia, ready to lead the parade to the field. A moment later I heard the sound of drums. The dancing began, with chanting and high-pitched non-chromatic singing. I was surrounded by feathers, tanned hides, colourful ribbons, moccasins, and headdresses. Everyone was bouncing to the rhythm, forming a line. They flowed into the open area in front of the stands and began travelling clockwise.

We held back as the dancers took the field, and then followed clumsily behind. I tried to figure out the bouncing rhythm, to step in harmony with the people in line. My colleagues seemed to be having no trouble with the beat, but I was lost. Suddenly, a hand took mine to lead me in the rhythm. A gentle hand, worn with farm work. I looked up to the face of the person whose hand held mine. It was Dennis, the husband of my patient Mavis, the woman who had called me the devil. Dennis, a respected Elder from Touchwood Hills, was one of the organizers of this event. We moved together towards the centre of the group. He didn't know that his presence in the hospital many months earlier had helped to guide my journey, but he did know he had rescued me from an embarrassing moment in the dance.

The patients that I see in the hospital and in community often speak in a conversational storytelling mode, reminding me of the circular Medicine Wheel. They may start with a story of something that happened when they were young, and this evolves into a lengthy exploration of their physical complaint. These stories often connect community, individual relationships, and the earth with traditional healing practices. "I put cabbage leaves soaked in milk on my leg, but it hasn't gotten better, so I came to see you, Doc." They may talk about spirituality and ceremonies. I have learned to be patient and listen. The circle has no beginning and no end. There is no power structure or dominance of one system over another—mental thinking does not trump emotions, physical does not trump spiritual—because everything is connected in a circle.

I was taught to think and speak in a linear tongue. One thing leads to another, step by step. For example, it seems clear to me that if you don't control your diabetes, you will suffer complications. This is linear, logical, focused, and ignores alternatives.[6] Experts say that linear thinkers excel at math, physics, and science. Many people who are interested in science become doctors; you have to excel at linear thinking to get through medical school, although the balance is changing. Over the span of my forty-year career, medical schools have fine-tuned an approach of teaching students to communicate through practising scenarios of difficult conversations. It takes time and experience to develop an empathetic manner; it requires facing one's own feelings. Physicians who have good insight into their strengths and limitations, who have developed empathy, and who have experience with difficult conversations tend to do better with patients. One thing that I learned over my career was the appreciation and welcoming of silence in medical interactions.

Even so, the physician often maintains a position of power, even domination. We hold the medical information, and we decide about when to communicate it. In a life-or-death situation, the patient may

---

6   This type of thinking has been ingrained in white settlers and is connected to the Doctrine of Discovery, a religious and legal concept long used to justify colonialism.

feel dominated, disrespected, and not in control, and this often triggers an overwhelming feeling of anger.

In short, many health providers talk too much. It's usually because we feel uncomfortable delivering the information we have to deliver, and we don't know how else to maintain our control and self-esteem. Of course, we may overlook the fact that the conversation is difficult for the patient. We generally try to act authoritative, since facing our own feelings and judgments requires vulnerability, and physicians are historically taught not to show vulnerability in front of patients.

The American Academy of Communication in Healthcare has documented the pattern of how physicians react when they encounter a difficult patient.[7] Almost universally, we feel incompetent, powerless, worthless, uncertain, stupid, inadequate, and humiliated. Driven by our feelings, we are likely to behave in one of three different ways. First, and most often, we use evasion, ignoring or talking over the patient in an effort to alleviate the physician's feeling of anxiety. This is the least harmful reaction. Second, our frustration about the patient's inability to take care of themselves can motivate us to lecture, threaten, or blame the patient. In the third, more dangerous, reaction, the physician expresses rage. This, obviously, can harm the patient. An example of this can be withholding narcotics from any patient in pain who appears to the physician to be manipulative. Through this behaviour, the physician can produce pain in the patient in order to justify the doctor's own anger.

When people from all over the world are surveyed about their relationship with their doctor, there is a range of responses. If the patient is healthy, they experience a positive relationship with their doctor. When a patient is sick, the relationship is different. In an American

---

7   Wendy Levinson, Cara S. Lesser, and Ronald M. Epstein, "Developing Physician Communication Skills for Patient-Centered Care," *Health Affairs* (Millwood) 29, no. 7 (July 2010):1,310–1,318, https://www.doi.org/10.1377/hlthaff.2009.0450.

study, only 40 percent of patients reported that their physicians had addressed their feelings or spent enough time with them.[8]

The pattern of physician domination applies to almost any patient or group of patients, whatever their background. In Saskatchewan, this comes with an overlay of colonialism—such as the often-unexamined assumption that Indigenous people are incapable of coping or behaving competently in industrial society.

The lesson that I learned from my first complaint letter was that I needed to examine my own role in communicating with patients. In the case of Mrs. D and her daughter, I felt resentful that I was being attacked. I had tried to help this young woman to the best of my ability, and in the end was accused of racism and entitlement. However, my letter of apology didn't mention my feelings of anger; I chose instead to cover up my personal feelings.

Looking back, I can see the behaviour that influenced Mrs. D's reaction. I made some classic mistakes: I used acronyms, I used technical terms, I used culturally inappropriate and offensive language. I insisted on a linear timeline in the death of her daughter. I tried to alleviate my own anxiety about her daughter's situation by talking over Mrs. D and acting Godlike.

I assumed that if I treated Mrs. D and her daughter with the professionalism that I use with non-Indigenous patients that I was treating them as equal. This is the classic definition of colourblindness—a type of racism that believes if you treat all people equally, then you are disregarding race, culture, and ethnicity. Although colourblindness is well-meaning, it has the unintended consequence of rejecting cultural

---

8 Kiara K. Spooner, Jason L. Salemi, Hamisu M. Salihu, and Roger J. Zoorob, "Disparities in Perceived Patient–Provider Communication Quality in the United States: Trends and Correlates," *Patient Education and Counseling* 99, no. 5 (May 2016), 844–854, https://doi.org/10.1016/j.pec.2015.12.007.

heritage. I suspect my attitude made Mrs. D feel like she was giving up her constitutionally protected rights: the right to be Indigenous. The right to be recognized with cultural differences that I was inadvertently trying to ignore.

Perhaps there was a lesson I could take from this distraught mother's path having crossed mine. I came to accept that I cannot assume anything about an Indigenous person's education level or their previous interactions with the health system. Nor can I assume awareness about their attitudes towards me as a representative of colonial authority. As I became more familiar with Indigenous cultural experience, I became less judgmental and began to examine my own racism.

I developed an interest in the concept of "two-eyed seeing." This is a technique that can be used to find a middle ground, or ethical space, between cultures. However, it is a difficult habit to develop. My friend and colleague Dr. JoLee Sasakamoose taught me about three things: two-eyed seeing, ethical space, and harmonizing. She referred me to the writings of Willie Ermine from First Nations University of Canada, who suggests that the *ethical space* is the space between two distinct views of the world—the circular Indigenous view and the linear Western institutions view.[9] Within this space, assumptions and history from each side need acknowledgement. As acknowledgement of two distinct views deepens, a middle space can be created. A non-Indigenous person cannot see the world from the Indigenous perspective but, with two-eyed seeing, I can make space for that perspective.

To get to the middle space, one must use one eye to understand the singular world consciousness of Western thought and the other eye to understand the circular patterns of Indigenous ways of knowing. These ways connect the spiritual with the physical world. This middle space

---

9   Willie Ermine, "The Ethical Space of Engagement," *Indigenous Law Journal* 6, no. 1 (2007), 193, https://jps.library.utoronto.ca/index.php/ilj/article/view/27669.

can create new currents of thought that embody two ways of seeing the world. Elder Albert Marshall from Mi'kmaq Nation says, "All people must learn two-eyed seeing so that knowledge of the physical is not separated from wisdom of the spiritual."[10]

Thanks to Mrs. D, I have embarked on the journey of learning the skill of seeing the world from an Indigenous perspective and from the perspective of settler society at the same time, to see the Medicine Wheel both in its original form and in the context of trans-generational trauma and the barriers and contradictions in the settler health care system. I began to explore the value of traditional lifestyles and the effects of Indigenous ceremonies to connect the spiritual with the physical, while continuing to explore aspects of my own racism.

I am cautious, however. There is a fallacy that the truth will be found somewhere in the middle between two opposing views. When there is a power imbalance, the middle ground is slanted. Two-eyed seeing tries to integrate the Indigenous view of the Medicine Wheel with the Western scientific view to facilitate cross-cultural communication. According to American anthropologist David Mandelbaum's ethnographic study of the Plains Cree, the concepts of communal property, sharing resources, ceremonies, rituals, and spirituality are integrated.[11] The concept of Indigenous ways of knowing is difficult for most linear thinkers schooled in Western thought patterns. A recently published book about Indigenous people who were taken to Europe to

---

10   Cheryl Bartlett, Murdena Marshall, Albert Marshall, and Marylin Iwama, "Integrative Science and Two-Eyed Seeing: Enriching the Discussion Framework for Healthy Communities" in *Ecosystems, Society and Health: Pathways through Diversity, Convergence and Integration*, ed. Lars K. Hallstrom, Nicholas Guehlstorf, and Margot Parkes (Montreal: McGill-Queen's University Press, 2015), 280–326.
11   David G. Mandelbaum, *The Plains Cree: An Ethnographic, Historical, and Comparative Study* (Saskatchewan: Canadian Plains Research Center, University of Regina, 1979).

"be civilized" in the 1500s provided me insight into the view from the other side. When the Indigenous people saw European culture, they were shocked by the gross economic inequities and cruelty towards the disadvantaged.[12] This perspective on our own Western culture is enlightening, and I continue to learn how to integrate the difference in the way we see the world. It goes beyond empathy and listening skills—it involves a completely different view of community relations. Finding the path to reconciliation requires stumbling over mistakes.

---

12   Caroline Dodds Pennock, *On Savage Shores: How Indigenous Americans Discovered Europe* (New York: Alfred A. Knopf, 2023).

A CRIME TO REFUSE TREATMENT

In my experience, there are some white people who grew up in Canada who will ask: Why do the Indians get all this free stuff? This question of Indigenous entitlement has spawned a lot of legal wrangling over many years between Ottawa and Indigenous Peoples; it encompasses more than income assistance and tax relief, and includes land rights, residential schools, blood quantum analysis, self-determination of governance, and the cultural revival of traditional Indigenous ways of knowing.

A related question: if the medicine chest clause was written into Treaty 6 at the last minute, to cover a specific area in the northern parts of Saskatchewan and Alberta, why do Indigenous people in other areas of Canada also get health care benefits from the federal government? The answer is complicated and not especially satisfying. The truth is that for generations after Alexander Morris promised the medicine chest, the people in Treaty 6 did not get much in the way of federal health care, nor did the people in southern Saskatchewan's Treaty 4 area (1874) or any other First Nation across Canada.

Then, around 1930, with a sustained tuberculosis epidemic threatening the settler population, Canada began to construct a separate and unequal Indian health care system. Finally, in about 1960, Indigenous people began to make legislative and legal gains (receiving the right to vote, for example). During this period, the medicine chest clause was tested in court. The court found that Indigenous people should receive government-funded health care services at no cost to them just like all other residents of Canada; at the same time, a federal commission recommended that Indigenous people receive health care services at the same standard as other citizens.

The European conquest of Turtle Island brought wave after wave of infectious disease to the original inhabitants. First it was smallpox, and then, in the late nineteenth century, it was tuberculosis, a respiratory disease that is often lethal. A medical survey developed in the late 1920s and focused on the Qu'Appelle Valley concluded that the tuberculosis epidemic in that region appeared in the early 1880s. By 1886, tuberculosis had killed an estimated ninety people out of every thousand in the local Indigenous population. Poverty, overcrowding, and malnutrition accelerated the spread of TB among Indigenous people. Tuberculosis remained the leading cause of death among Indigenous people in Saskatchewan until the early 1950s, rates roughly twenty times as high as those seen in the general population.[1]

The first quarter of the twentieth century also saw the spread of high rates of tuberculosis to the settler and immigrant populations in North America. Governments began to construct special care centres for tuberculosis patients, focusing on non-pharmaceutical measures

---

[1] Joanne M. Hader, "The Effect of Tuberculosis on the Indians of Saskatchewan: 1926–1965," graduate thesis, University of Saskatchewan, 1990; "Tuberculosis History in Canada, from 1867 to 2020," TB in Focus, https://www.tbinfocus.ca/tb-history-in-canada/.

since medical science had not yet discovered antibiotics. The first "sanatorium" in Canada opened in 1897 in Gravenhurst, Ontario. By 1938, Canada had sixty-one sanatoria and over nine thousand beds for the treatment of TB. Saskatchewan built three sanatoria: at Fort Qu'Appelle (1917), Saskatoon (1925), and Prince Albert (1930). They were open, at least in theory, to Indigenous and non-Indigenous patients.

Treatment of TB at the sanatorium relied on rest, good nutrition, fresh air, and isolation. In her book *Indian Hospitals in Canada*, Maureen Lux describes the treatment of Indigenous patients: "Rambunctious children were often physically restrained in their beds, or by plaster casts on both legs. Patients in hospitals far from home often did not understand the language, and struggled to understand their treatment, if it was explained to them. Caregivers, many overworked and underpaid, took out their frustrations on patients. Children without family nearby were particularly vulnerable."[2] So, in addition to residential schools, children were taken from their homes to be placed in TB sanatoriums. When I imagine children put into body casts to keep them at rest, as a supposed cure for TB, I get nauseated.

The high rates of illness and death from TB generated an ongoing conversation in the Canadian news media. The continued very high rates of illness and death among Indigenous people caused widespread alarm about patterns of transmission. Some in the settler population considered the Indians to be the cause of the disease; it was believed that contact with them would allow TB to leak into non-Indigenous communities. This resulted not only in social isolation, but it also influenced public health and government policy: because Indigenous patients were considered reckless and irresponsible in their management of TB, they should legally be separated from the non-Indigenous population.

---

2   Maureen Lux, "Indian Hospitals in Canada," The Canadian Encyclopedia online, July 17, 2017, https://www.thecanadianencyclopedia.ca/en/article/indian-hospitals-in-canada.

Indigenous communities were aware of the death rate from tuberculosis and concerned about the barriers they were facing in seeking treatment. In 1928, a group of Elders from the Pasqua First Nation in the Qu'Appelle Valley travelled to Ottawa to advocate for the recognition of the Treaty 6 medicine chest clause as a baseline commitment to all First Nations. They also argued that they should not be excluded from community hospitals.[3] But instead of helping to integrate the existing hospitals, the Department of Indian Affairs began to develop separate hospitals and fund religious organizations to treat Indigenous people separately from the non-Indigenous population. In 1936, eight years after the Pasqua Elders petitioned Ottawa, the Fort Qu'Appelle Indian Hospital was established. It was used mainly as a sanatorium for the treatment of TB.

The actions of one physician in southern Saskatchewan had wide-reaching implications for the treatment of tuberculosis. Dr. Robert George Ferguson graduated from medical school in Winnipeg in 1916 and was appointed acting superintendent of Fort San, the new sanatorium at Fort Qu'Appelle, in 1917. As the only doctor at Fort San, he was on call twenty-four hours a day and lived in a house beside the sanatorium with his family. He was tireless in his advocacy for the treatment of TB, irrespective of race.

One of the barriers to TB treatment was its high cost in the early part of the twentieth century. The average length of stay for patients at the sanatorium was twelve months; the fee for such a stay, in the order of $2,000, was more than most people would earn in a year. Ferguson became a strong advocate of free treatment for TB and was a supporter of the Saskatchewan Anti-Tuberculosis League, which raised money to provide treatment for patients in need. The league

---

3   Constance Backhouse, *Colour-Coded: A Legal History of Racism in Canada, 1900–1950* (Toronto: University of Toronto Press, 1999).

lobbied successfully for legislation that by 1929 provided treatment of TB at no cost to the patient.[4] This early milestone in the development of Saskatchewan's medical care system preceded the adoption of universal hospital insurance, through the 1940s and '50s, and universal medical insurance in 1962.

Dr. Ferguson undertook one of the first clinical trials of TB treatment with a vaccination program in 1933. The Bacillus Calmette–Guérin vaccine (BCG) had first gone into medical use in 1921. Children born to Dr. Ferguson's Indigenous patients in Fort Qu'Appelle were vaccinated at birth with BCG, while a control group of children born on reserve with a midwife did not receive the vaccine. He collected data on the development of TB in the two groups over time and found that the incidence of TB was five times greater in the unvaccinated group, results that he reported at the National Association for the Prevention of Tuberculosis in Great Britain. His data showed that vaccination of children reduced the rate of TB infection.

Ferguson has been described as patronizing and colonialist in some accounts; some have viewed the Qu'Appelle Valley TB trial as an experiment on Indigenous children. In other narratives, he is portrayed as a compassionate man who treated his patients as equals and, in turn, they respected him. In 1935, the File Hills First Nation gave him what he considered the greatest honour of his life: recognition as the honorary Chief Great White Physician Muskeke-O-Kemacan.[5] He retired after thirty-one years at Fort San, and he died a few decades later in 1964. Many of my elderly patients have told me stories about Ferguson's generation of prairie doctors who devoted their lives to the fundamentals

---

4   G. Dudley Barnett, "Tuberculosis Control," The Encyclopedia of Saskatchewan online, https://esask.uregina.ca/entry/tuberculosis_control.jsp.
5   C. Stuart Houston and Merle Massie, *36 Steps on the Road to Medicare: Why Saskatchewan Led the Way* (Montreal: McGill-Queens University Press, 2002), 59.

of medical practice, visiting patients on farms and reserves through the 1930s and 1940s.

The segregated Indian hospitals were constructed by means of what was becoming a relatively large federal budget for Indigenous health care. Starting in the 1920s, the Liberal government of William Lyon MacKenzie King began to build Indian hospitals, hire Indian Health Service nurses and doctors, provide medicines, and implement public health initiatives. A report from parliamentary committee hearings on the Indian Act says that in 1946 spending on health care for First Nations people was $2.3 million, approximately the same as the budget for residential schools.[6]

Unfortunately, the Indian hospitals incorporated some of the features of the residential schools, and as of 1953, confinement to an Indian hospital was no longer voluntary. An amendment to the Indian Act that year, called the Indian Health Regulations, made it a crime for Indigenous people to refuse to see a doctor or go to hospital, or to leave hospital before being discharged. The RCMP was empowered to arrest patients and returned them to hospital or send them to jail.[7]

The segregated Indian hospitals were still alive in memory among some of my patients after I returned to Canada. One day at a clinic in the Touchwood Hills, I opened the consulting room door for Dorothy, a calm seventy-six-year-old who told me she was afraid of doctors and hospitals and then related the story behind the fear. She had attended a residential school as a girl, became sick as a result, and was sent to the Indian hospital at Fort Qu'Appelle. Like most of the children and

---

6   From John Leslie, "Assimilation, Integration or Termination? The Development of Canadian Indian Policy, 1943–1963," doctoral thesis, Carleton University, Ottawa, 1999, https://doi.org/10.22215/etd/1999-04189. On page 120 of this thesis, Leslie reviews the findings from the Special Joint Committee Hearings on the Indian Act that met between 1946 and 1948.

7   Lux, "Indian Hospitals in Canada."

adults sent there, she was diagnosed with tuberculosis. A male orderly frequently approached her bed in the night to fondle her. This left her with a fear of hospitals. When she was released and returned to her family, her grandmother accompanied her through many sweats in the Sweat Lodge. They healed together. The Elders told her that people would want to know about her time at the hospital and at school, and she would have to learn to answer their questions. Despite her healing, she still doesn't like hospitals. Dorothy began to cry as she told me her story. I hugged her and thanked her for opening up, yet I could not convince her to go to the hospital when she was sick.

The 1940s and '50s saw the birth of modern Indigenous activism in Canada. By 1957, when national hospital insurance was implemented for all Canadians,[8] the federal Indian Health Services branch decided to quietly divest itself of its twenty-six hospitals. In 1962, the Chiefs from Treaty 6 area (Poundmaker, Sweetgrass, Onion Lake, and Little Pine) submitted a protest to the Indian Health Services branch, requesting recognition of their treaty rights for health care.[9] As Indian hospitals closed and Canadian provinces started up their Medicare programs, Ottawa created a list of Non-Insured Health Benefits (NIHB) for

---

8   "The Hospital Insurance and Diagnostic Services Act (HIDS) is a statute passed by the Parliament of Canada in 1957 that reimbursed one-half of provincial and territorial costs for hospital and diagnostic services administered under provincial and territorial health insurance programs....By January 1, 1961, all ten provinces were enlisted. The federal funding was coupled with terms and conditions borrowed from the Saskatchewan Hospital Services Plan, introduced in 1947 as the first universal hospital insurance program in North America." From "Hospital Insurance and Diagnostic Services Act," Wikipedia, https://en.wikipedia.org/wiki/Hospital_Insurance_and_Diagnostic_Services_Act.

9   The Glassco Commission was a wide-ranging investigation into the Government of Canada's organization and methods of operation. See Mélanie Brunet, "The Glassco Commission and Its Repercussions," *Out of the Shadows: The Civil Law Tradition in the Department of Justice Canada, 1868–2000*, Government of Canada, February 2, 2023, https://www.justice.gc.ca/eng/rp-pr/other-autre/civil/place4.html.

Indigenous people to supplement the basket of services covered by provincial medical insurance. This included coverage for drugs, equipment, and transportation for medical care.

The Indian hospital in North Battleford finally closed in 1971, after much wrangling with government bureaucrats.[10] The Indian hospital in Fort Qu'Appelle transitioned to the Touchwood File Hills Qu'Appelle Tribal Council in the 1990s and was replaced by All Nations' Healing Hospital in 2004. In 2018, former patients of Indian hospitals across Canada filed a $1.1 billion class-action lawsuit against the federal government, seeking financial compensation and a formal acknowledgement of the government's negligence in the operation of those hospitals.[11] At the time of this writing, no measurable progress has been made to resolve these claims against Indian hospitals. In the meantime, after the death of Joyce Echaquan in 2020, an Atikamekw organization has petitioned for Joyce's Principle.[12] This principle advocates that Indigenous people be guaranteed the right to equitable access to health care without discrimination.

The Section 73 amendment of the Indian Act (1876) in the 1970s delineated the authority of the federal government to prevent and address the spread of disease on reserves.[13] The negotiation of post-Confederation treaties from Ontario to British Columbia often included a discussion

---

10 Maureen K. Lux, *Separate Beds: A History of Indian Hospitals in Canada, 1920s–1980s* (Toronto: University of Toronto Press, 2016).

11 Lauren Pelley, "$1.1B Class-Action Lawsuit Filed on Behalf of Former 'Indian Hospital' Patients," CBC News, January 30, 2018, https://www.cbc.ca/news/canada/toronto/indian-hospital-class-action-1.4508659.

12 Council of the Atikamekw of Manawan and the council de la nation Atikamekw, "Joyce's Principle," November 2020, https://principedejoyce.com/sn_uploads/principe/Joyce_s_Principle_brief___Eng.pdf.

13 Section 73(f) of the Indian Act gives government power to make regulations "to prevent, mitigate and control the spread of diseases on reserves, whether or not the diseases are infectious or communicable."

about health care provisions, especially since Indigenous Peoples had watched smallpox and starvation destroy their populations. It was only in Treaty 6, however, that the promises were written down in the form of a medicine chest clause. In 1996 the Supreme Court of Canada (*Regina v. Badger*) finally ruled that oral histories and consent are, in fact, part of the Government of Canada's treaty obligations, confirming that the promises made to Treaty 6 should apply to other treaty areas.

+ + +

Tuberculosis is still a threat to First Nations health in the twenty-first century, despite the implementation of population-based interventions. The introduction of infant vaccination with BCG, public health contact tracing in communities, and effective drug treatment have helped, but the cases have recently increased. Indigenous people in Canada have nearly three hundred times the risk of getting TB than non-Indigenous, representing nearly 20 percent of all TB cases in the country.[14] Among people with tuberculosis in Canada, 70 percent are First Nations, Métis, or recent immigrants.[15]

With all diseases and conditions, and with all populations, compliance with treatment regimens is one of the biggest issues of concern that we face as physicians. The primary treatment for TB in Saskatchewan is DOT (directly observed therapy), the World Health Organization standard for doctors in working with infected populations. The requirement, quite simply, is for the patient to stand in front of a health care

---

14 Sarah Hick, "The Enduring Plague: How Tuberculosis in Canadian Indigenous Communities Is Emblematic of a Greater Failure in Healthcare Equality," *Journal of Epidemiology and Global Health* 9, no. 2 (June 2019): 89–92, https://doi.org/10.2991/jegh.k.190314.002.

15 Bruce F. Tapiéro and Valerie Lamarre, "Tuberculosis in Canada: Global View and New Challenges," *Paediatrics & Child Health* 8, no. 3 (March 2003), 139–140, https://doi.org/10.1093/pch/8.3.139

worker or a trusted community member who watches them swallow their pills. This has diminished the frequency of treatment failure in Indigenous populations, but it has not ended the pattern of epidemics. An outbreak was declared in Northern Saskatchewan First Nations in 2021.[16] The medical officer of the Northern Inter-Tribal Health Authority was reported as saying the most powerful form of prevention of tuberculosis would be to invest in housing[17]—inadequate housing being, in his view, the root cause of the disease's spread. Housing as the cause of an infectious disease? Yes, because TB spreads in crowded settings. Medical science focuses on how an organism infects the human body, replicates, and transmits to others. Sophisticated pharma laboratories design drugs to treat the organism and eradicate its spread. The clash between science and public policy and public health is a nuance of the medicine chest clause that requires further discussion.

In addition to TB, other epidemics have devastated Indigenous populations. During my career, and especially since 2000, we have seen the rise of new epidemics driven by adverse social conditions among Indigenous people. HIV infection related to intravenous drug use has been particularly deadly. Among other risks, HIV poses a high risk of reactivation of latent TB and rapid progression of new infections with TB.

A Canada-wide survey in 2012 found that "new HIV diagnoses per year remained essentially constant for all other provinces except for the Prairies, where rates increased two-fold driven by new infections in the

---

16 Dayne Patterson, "Tuberculosis Outbreaks Declared in Northern First Nations Communities," CBC News, October 10, 2021, https://www.cbc.ca/news/canada/saskatchewan/tuberculosis-outbreaks-declared-in-northern-first-nations-communities-1.6206617.

17 Dr. Nnamdi Ndubuka, medical health officer for the Northern Inter-Tribal Health Authority in Saskatchewan, quoted Zak Vescera, "Time to invest in ending tuberculosis in Sask., doctors say," *Saskatoon StarPhoenix*, March 24, 2022, https://thestarphoenix.com/news/saskatchewan/time-to-invest-in-ending-tuberculosis-in-sask-doctors-say.

province of Saskatchewan."[18] As we surveyed the population, we found out that Saskatchewan's new HIV cases were mainly in the Indigenous community. The medicine chest clause in the treaties, originally signed to treat epidemics, became even more important.

---

18   Robert S. Hogg, Katherine Heath, Viviane D. Lima, Bohdan Nosyk, Steve Kanters, Evan Wood, Thomas Kerr, and Julio S. G. Montaner, "Disparities in the Burden of HIV/AIDS in Canada," *PLOS ONE* 7, no. 11 (12), e47260, https://doi.org/10.1371/journal.pone.0047260; correction published in *PLOS ONE* 13, no. 12 (December 6, 2018), e0209045, https://doi.org/10.1371/journal.pone.0209045.

AS LONG AS THAT SUN SHINES

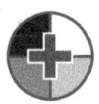

After three years of working in the Saskatchewan health care system, in hospital and in my private office, I'd had direct experience of working with Indigenous patients and began recognizing last names: some came from nature, like Crow, Bird, Wolf, Eagle, Bear, Badger, Whitehawk, and Buffalo; some names were Scottish, like MacKenzie, Campbell, and McKay; and others were French, like Desjarlais, Favel, LaPlante, and Pelletier...But I had no idea where these names came from or how they were related. I had read about the historical and social forces that kept most Indigenous people in a powerless state. I had a few cordial, if distant, working relationships with Indigenous nurses and care aides at the hospital, but essentially zero contact with anything that could be called an Indigenous community.

I felt I was not truly connecting, and as a result, I wasn't understanding what I was seeing.

Why were so many Indigenous patients landing in hospital, especially when access to hospital was often difficult? Approximately 17 percent of Saskatchewan's population, about 188,000 people, identified as

Indigenous in 2021—perhaps a third of them in the cities, a third on rural reserves, mainly in the south, and a third in remote villages in Saskatchewan's vast north. Yet I would estimate that more than 30 percent of the patients in the hospital during my years at Regina General were Indigenous—overrepresented in hospital on a population basis.

More troubling was the high rate of terminal disease that I was seeing. Uncontrolled diabetes, high rates of dialysis, poorly treated hypertension, chronic lung disease, heart attacks in middle-aged people, higher rates of amputations—all diseases and conditions that are preventable with good, comprehensive medical care. The frequency of these conditions exceeded the inner-city problems I had seen in the United States. In the US, African American people, many of whom live in the inner city, experience poorer health than people who are white. Scholarly articles point to economic and social conditions to explain the differences. Unemployment, poverty, low rates of home ownership, smoking, obesity, and sedentary lifestyle all contribute to the higher death rate.[1] The public health community has long recognized these factors, calling them social determinants of health. It is a matter of life and death from a social justice perspective, which increases the chances of illness and premature death.[2] Around the world, such inequalities have given rise to outrage, protest, lobbying, and the creation of complex social programs, and yet the inequalities persist.

---

1   National Center for Chronic Disease Prevention and Health Promotion (US), Centers for Disease Control and Prevention (US), and Office of the Associate Director for Communications, "African American Health: Creating Equal Opportunity for Health," CDC *Vital Signs*, May 2, 2017, https://stacks.cdc.gov/view/cdc/45439.
2   From a landmark report aimed at understanding health inequities from a social justice perspective. World Health Organization Commission on Social Determinants of Health, "Closing the Gap in a Generation: Health Equity through Action on the Social Determinants of Health," Geneva, World Health Organization, 2008, https://apps.who.int/iris/bitstream/handle/10665/43943/9789241563703_eng.pdf.

In Canada, Indigenous people are hospitalized 2.6 times more frequently than the non-Indigenous population,[3] and I was seeing plenty of these admissions in Regina. Hospital beds are expensive, and they are scarce. The Regina General Hospital and Pasqua Hospital in Regina have only around 250 medical beds between them;[4] they are the closest points of acute care for perhaps 250,000 people in the city and surrounding area. As tertiary care centres, they provide specialized acute care, beyond the level of community hospitals, for another 250,000 rural people. Most complex admissions to hospital are handled by the Internal Medicine service, of which I am a member. People who come into hospital tend to fall into categories: the frail elderly, people with chronic disease who are not coping at home, people with heart disease, people who have chronic lung disease from smoking, people with acute infectious disease, and newly diagnosed cancer. Indigenous patients are found in all categories.

In the United States, many low-income people can't afford to see a doctor, an often-cited reason for the relatively poor health of African Americans. We have universal health insurance in Canada—nobody is denied access to basic care on a financial basis—and yet I was seeing a constant flow of Indigenous people with end-stage chronic diseases in my outpatient office and in hospital. I pondered the puzzle, turning over the pieces in my head like a Rubik's Cube.

+ + +

3   Gisèle Carrière, Evelyne Bougie, Dafna Kohen, Michelle Rotermann, and Claudia Sanmartin, "Acute Care Hospitalization by Indigenous Identity, Canada, 2006 through 2008," *Health Reports* 27, no. 8 (August 17, 2016), 3–11, https://pubmed.ncbi.nlm.nih.gov/27532620/.
4   Medical beds are those allocated to patients admitted by family and Internal Medicine physicians; the rest of the hospital beds in Regina are allocated to ICU, surgery, cardiology, neurology, cancer care, obstetrics, and pediatrics.

As I drive out of the doctors' parking lot at the hospital late on a sunny afternoon in October 2015, the swinging gate opens. I flash my hospital badge over the electronic lock. A three-storey apartment building shadows the exit. Out of the corner of my eye I notice a pair of shoes protruding from the edge of the large rectangular trash container at the end of the one-lane alley that connects the parking lot to the street. I don't want to stop and stare, but I proceed past slowly. A lumberjack shirt and a man's head appear as the scavenger jackknifes to a precarious upright position. Dumpster diving, in Regina and other Canadian cities, is an occupation that provides a sort of living for those with agility, persistence, and an eye for value.

When I get home, most of the October leaves are either lying on the ground or trapped in gutters around the house. My father announces that we have had a visitor and will have a second one within the hour. During the day he hired a young Indigenous man who was wandering the neighbourhood on foot with a ladder to clean the gutters.

"Only twenty dollars, cash," he tells me.

The second visitor is the health care economist Greg Marchildon. Greg, a former student of Dad's, regularly visits to discuss his work and other things. Greg has expert knowledge of international health care trends as well as about the establishment of Medicare in Canada. His relationship with my father extends beyond social policy discussions into friendship. Greg lost his father at an early age, so my dad is like a father to him, offering support and advice about love, child rearing, and career decisions.

During this evening's visit, I am introduced again to the centuries of history during which colonists and settlers have accumulated an enormous debt to the original occupants of this land.

"In my work," I say to Greg, "I often find myself treating diseases that have progressed so far that I have little to offer. These are conditions that were labeled as 'end-stage' when I was in medical school. How can

Indigenous people appear in the ER with so many end-stage diseases when we have a single-payer medical system in Canada that covers everyone? They have had access to care all along, without having to worry about their ability to pay."

I am expressing my frustration with the health system, and my own personal sense of helplessness as a physician who is trying to help. I am excited to hear his thoughts, given his expertise.

"The medicine chest," says Greg. "A promise made and broken. The first hospital in Saskatchewan territory was opened up by the Sisters of Charity in 1860, at Île-à-la-Crosse in the far north. The Mounted Police had hospitals at their forts, starting with Fort Walsh in the Cypress Hills in 1875. By 1876, when Treaty 6 was signed, the Chiefs were ready to demand medical services for their people, to treat the white man's diseases. They negotiated this in addition to existing provisions included in previous treaties for land, schools, and food. That's how we got the medicine chest clause."

I reflect on how Treaty 6 was signed. Alexander Morris, the Treaty 6 commissioner, pledged that this was a serious commitment: "What I trust and hope we will do is not for today or tomorrow only; what I promise and what I believe and hope you will take, is to last as long as that sun shines and yonder river *flows*."[5] Unfortunately, the care that was provided from the medicine chest for the first fifty years was minimal; this was followed by the segregated care system, where treatment facilities were separate and unequal.

My father chimes in: "Jarol, when I was growing up in Briercrest and my dad was working labouring jobs to supply food for our family, he worked side-by-side with Indians." Although my father was a

---

5   Alexander Morris, *The Treaties of Canada with the Indians of Manitoba and the North-West Territories: Including the Negotiations on Which They Were Based, and Other Information Relating Thereto* (Saskatoon: Fifth House Publishers, 1991), 202.

big-hearted and empathetic man, he was also ninety-five years old and had not learned to be politically correct in his nomenclature. "Provincial Medicare arrived in the early sixties. It was supposed to provide access to health care for everyone, without regard to cost."

I ask, "Did it make any difference to Indigenous people and Métis?"

Greg reminds me: "When provincial Medicare was started in the early sixties, Indigenous people were considered residents of Saskatchewan. The Saskatchewan Health Plan covers everyone in the province, including Indigenous people.[6]

"However," Greg continues, "the universal health insurance didn't create any new programs or changes in jurisdiction. The federal government still had responsibility for registered treaty status members, on and off reserves. There was a health agency attached to the federal Department of Indian Affairs, and it seems the main result of Medicare was to encourage the federal government to back away from its responsibilities and the medicine chest clause, and to simply make payments to the provinces for whatever services Indigenous people could locate in provincial hospitals and clinics."

I reply: "As a young student at the University of Regina, I remember hearing about the Chiefs' organizations that were formed in the 1970s, such as the National Indian Brotherhood and Assembly of First Nations. These activists were vocal in pressing for better health care, among other things to help their people. The federal government conducted a national survey.[7] It found that Indigenous infant mortality was

---

6   All Indigenous people have status as "Indian" as defined by subsections 6(1) and 6(2) of the Indian Act (1876). It applies to both those who signed treaties and those who did not. An Indigenous person can also be non-status—for example, someone from the Sixties Scoop who cannot access their parents' status to prove eligibility. A non-status Indigenous person is covered under provincial Medicare, like the rest of the non-Indigenous population.

7   Kue Young, "Indian Health Services in Canada: A Sociohistorical Perspective,"...

ten times the national rate, the average age of death was forty-one years, 37 percent of families had no secure housing, and 98 percent had no sewer or water. Nobody on reserve had a telephone to call for medical help. The report recommended infrastructure development and proper clinics to replace on-reserve nursing stations. Even with this evidence, there was almost no action."

"If those recommendations had been followed," Greg says, "the subsequent drain on provincial and federal health care budgets from epidemic disease would have been reduced."

Housing. Clean water. Telephones. On-reserve clinics. Greg's words stay with me for weeks as I work in the hospitals and my private office and witness the social issues that surround me. I began hearing about paths to reconciliation but didn't know what it meant. I am only a doctor with an ability to diagnose disease and treat the sick. I am not a social worker, nor a politician.

A few months later, while I'm out on an errand, I get a call on my mobile phone from Dr. Stu Skinner. He's the infectious disease specialist whom I met in the hospital shortly after I arrived in Regina. I don't know him well, but I've enjoyed working with him. Stu is about forty years old, thin, athletic, with sandy brown hair and a boyish face. He gives me advice about how and when to prescribe antibiotics for the multiple infections that I manage, and he shares knowledge of local infection trends based on his work in the hospital laboratories. I'm in awe of his expertise, and I respect his humility and non-judgmental caring attitude.

We both know that the treatment of infection is related to the underlying social factors that produced the disease. Through our multiple interactions looking at the charts of hospitalized patients, he has realized that I understand this connection.

...*Social Science & Medicine* 18, no. 3 (February 1984) 257–64, https://doi.org/10.1016/0277-9536(84)90088-1.

Today, his voice is gentle but firm in its intent. "Look, I have an idea that needs some work. I want to start a program to bring medical services to the reserve, and you'd be a great addition to the team. I'm starting right away. I've got a meeting at the Touchwood Hills Tribal Agency. Next Tuesday. Do you want to come?"

I'm already aware of some of the background behind this trip; the rising rates of HIV and Hepatitis C in our patient population are trends that are a regular agenda item in our medical staff meetings at Regina General. Stu has been working for the past five years with Indigenous people in Northern Saskatchewan to stem the causes of these epidemics. Now he wants to expand to the southern part of the province, to send a team to reserves to address chronic disease in its early stages. I scroll through my mental calendar to check for scheduling conflicts and immediately agree. "I'll meet you at the hospital parking lot on Tuesday at 8:00 a.m.," he says, buoyant and hopeful.

Suddenly I have become someone who has chosen to contribute to an Indigenous community in an intentional way. I'm excited about the opportunity. As it turns out, I'm also on my way to entering difficult terrain where I'll be reminded, in new ways, about the face of white privilege and the barriers to providing health care across cultures.

STRANGERS IN THE TOUCHWOOD HILLS

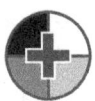

The project started slowly in 2016, while we considered how to proceed with the logistics of taking a health care team to a cluster of reserves in central Saskatchewan. We were committed to helping, and we understood the need to engage with communities both physically and spiritually. We had adapted the project name, "Wellness Wheel," from Medicine Wheel, to show our desire to enhance every dimension of the human experience.

The most urgent motivator was the deepening epidemic of HIV among the Indigenous people in Saskatchewan, combined with an epidemic of Hepatitis C. From 2007 through 2016, the rate of HIV infections in Saskatchewan was generally more than twice that of Canada as a whole.[1] Of the total Saskatchewan population infected with HIV, Indigenous people made up between 70 and 80 percent. Of all HIV

---

[1] Ministry of Health Population Health Branch, Government of Saskatchewan, *HIV Prevention and Control Report*, 2016, https://saskatchewan.ca/health.

cases diagnosed in Saskatchewan, 45 percent were Indigenous women.[2] Hepatitis C rates were also increasing; over 64 percent of our Hepatitis C patient population was Indigenous, and 55 percent of those infected with Hepatitis C were also living with HIV.

The medical staff at Regina General Hospital had been debating the best response to these epidemics for months. We asked ourselves, Can we provide better treatment for the Indigenous population? Can we protect people who use drugs from complications such as HIV and Hepatitis C? We recognized that isolation on the reserve, barriers to primary care, barriers to testing, barriers to seeing specialists, and transportation barriers were contributing to poor health outcomes. Stu Skinner was already familiar and comfortable with travelling to communities; for him, it was an easy decision to expand his efforts into a new geographic area. He also knew that individual diseases don't happen in a vacuum, and that uncontrolled diabetes, like drug use, occurs in a social context.

Stu had firm ideas about self-determination. He knew that we needed to consult people on reserve from the start, to get their guidance on how we could meet their needs. We felt confident that we were on the right track after we left our meeting with Valerie Desjarlais at the Touchwood Agency Tribal Council headquarters, about ninety minutes north from Regina. Val, a member of the Kawacatoose First Nation, was energetic and enthusiastic. Her position as health director for the Tribal Council would provide us with the connections and guidance we needed to engage with the various Council-operated health centres.

For that first meeting, Stu parked near the door of the Tribal Council's health centre, shared with the Muskowekwan First Nation bingo hall. We watched a middle-aged, dark-haired woman dressed in a flowing skirt and T-shirt approach us with a huge smile. She led us in,

---

2   Personal communication with Dr. Alexander Wong, infectious disease specialist in Regina, SK, November 8, 2018.

and we sat in the lunchroom while she told us her story. Val was passionate about her people after overcoming her own struggles. She had recovered from alcohol and drug addiction in her youth and wanted to give back to her community. She had attended night school to obtain a degree in human justice from University of Regina, and she had trained in working with individuals with post-traumatic stress disorder at Red River College in Winnipeg, Manitoba. While attending school in Regina, she helped to establish a street outreach program counselling sexually exploited women and sex workers. She spoke with great energy but also with humility.

The Touchwood Agency Tribal Council (TATC) had formed in 1999 to pool the federal government resources that were available to four neighbouring reserves. One of its challenges was to deal with the federal ministry responsible for meeting Canada's political, constitutional, legal, and treaty obligations to those the federal government identify as being Indigenous. Like many government agencies, the ministry had gone through an accelerating round of restructuring and renaming. At this time, in 2016 when Wellness Wheel started, it was known as Indigenous and Northern Affairs Canada (INAC) and by 2017 it was then split in two: Crown-Indigenous Relations and Northern Affairs Canada (CIRNAC) and Indigenous Services Canada (ISC).

The Tribal Council's governance structure made it responsible for economic and job development, justice, housing, education, and health. Val, as health program manager, helped to obtain band council resolutions that supported the proposed clinics. This would allow us to offer clinical care in the local health centres on four reserves—Muskowekwan, Kawacatoose, Day Star, and George Gordon First Nation—and in this capacity she was instrumental in providing us access to the staff in the health centres on our clinic days.

We started our program of visits within a few weeks. The home care nurses or diabetic educators at the health centres would identify patients who needed care and put them on our list. They faxed this list to the city on the day before our clinic day. In the beginning, if there were ten patients on the list, perhaps three would show up. Care was uncoordinated and not documented. We made it up as we went along, and as we identified missing pieces of the care continuum, we filled in the gaps.

Stu Skinner and I normally travelled as a pair. After a few months, Val carved out a small budget from the federal health programming funds that she was authorized to spend, and we hired a part-time nurse. Susanne Nicolay had worked as an HIV services coordinator in Regina, and in her new role with Wellness Wheel she worked to coordinate patient visits, plan our time, and communicate with each health centre. Her role was invaluable.

We felt good when we were able to recruit two additional physicians to provide primary care and treat diabetes, hypertension, and infection: Dr. Thanh Luu, tall with straight dark hair, and Dr. Megan Clark, short and blonde, both of whom worked at the Family Medicine Unit in Regina, also joined us. These doctors took one day per month of vacation from their regular jobs, and we rotated their assignments to treat patients on reserve. They were particularly interested in the vulnerable populations who had no access to care. Both of them were caring, compassionate, and good communicators. They were instantly likeable people.

Soon after we started visiting the Touchwood Hills, a sixty-five-year-old patient came to the health centre on reserve with diabetes. She needed refills on her medication. As she was leaving the consultation room, she mentioned that she was having vaginal bleeding with clots. Vaginal bleeding after menopause is a red flag, so Dr. Luu asked the patient if she could do an examination. The patient agreed. We found the instruments we needed, and the patient lay down on the exam table. During the speculum exam, there was significant bleeding.

Dr. Luu was especially concerned when she saw a larger fungating mass on the patient's cervix. The immediate concern was for advanced cervical cancer.

We called Regina and got the patient an appointment with a gynecologist for the next day. How long had she had this mass? With no regular medical services available on reserve, she had never had a full physical assessment.

From the exam, there was blood everywhere. We dropped the paper drape and bed sheets into a garbage can and cleaned and sanitized the exam table. We cleaned the blood off the floor and tossed the cleaning cloths in the garbage can as well. We felt confident that we had done what needed to be done. But as we were leaving the building, ready to get in the car to drive back to Regina, one of the health centre employees stopped us.

With a stern look she said: "You can't put your garbage in our garbage can. It is not our responsibility to dispose of your mess."

We looked at each other. We hadn't thought that the reserve infrastructure was so limited that they had no garbage collection. Dressed in our winter parkas, hats, gloves, and boots, we returned to the rear of the health clinic and collected the green garbage bags. We put them in the trunk of our car and drove them to Regina for disposal at the hospital.

As it turned out, Indigenous communities do operate a garbage pickup service. In the local Health Director's view, however, this was our garbage, and not a problem for the clinic to deal with. We had chosen to come on to the reserve, and in her view we were imposing costs on the community and the Tribal Council. To leave our trash behind added insult to injury.

From our perspective, in that moment, the trash was theirs, since the blood we mopped up was from one of their residents on reserve. Technically, however, she was right. The operation of our clinic created an issue around the disposal of human material. There is always a risk that fresh blood may contain Hepatitis, HIV, or other dangerous contaminants. In the hospital setting, blood-soaked materials go into bags and then into a special container labeled *Contaminated*. The hospital employs a specialized company to collect and dispose of these materials through a provincially permitted process. This health centre had none of that, except for plastic bins that collected used needles from the pediatric vaccination program.

In the end, as Wellness Wheel and the local staff achieved mutual respect, we reached a long-term compromise on the handling of waste. "Red Bin" contaminated waste would go to Regina with the medical team for appropriate disposal; regular waste, the large majority of our volumes, would be deposited in the bins behind the reserve clinics for pickup by local community contractors.

Despite our meetings with Val, we had not established any clear delineation of roles. The clinic staff saw us as behaving like helicopter parents—hovering, stepping in to make decisions, not collaborating with the local health team to solve concerns or problems, taking away their ability to direct us in their centre and community—classic demonstrations of colonialist attitudes. The nurses and support staff worked on the reserve, and many of them also lived within the community. We only catapulted into their world every couple of weeks. Among their concerns was the fact that our drive-by diagnosis would sometimes leave them to provide a drug or a treatment that they didn't understand and would add to their responsibilities for patient care between clinical care visits.

Before long, we pulled back somewhat, adopting a less dominant role during our visits. We were learning how to build respectful partnership in health care. We reassured the local nurses that our medical, nursing, and pharmaceutical support would be available to them after we left. We used our personal mobile phones for these communications. To reduce the impact of our clinics on local staff, we carried in our equipment and medical supplies—stethoscopes, blood-pressure cuffs, otoscope to check ears, thermometer, glucometer, over-the-counter medications, supplies for drawing blood, and plastic travelling bins for storage.

Throughout 2017, we held between three and four clinics per month for an annual total of forty-five per year, all of it outside the federal government's health services funding process. Val and the Tribal Council paid our transportation costs and travel time for our team members, but up to four hours each clinic day was unpaid. As a physician, I was able to bill the Saskatchewan Medical Services Branch on a fee-for-service basis for every patient that I encountered. This was not a big money-maker; many patients did not show up for their appointments. But this was a start-up program, and like any start-up we had the right attitude: we had a vision, we had commitment, we were willing to start small, and we were willing to engage the community. I had confidence that it would grow.

The treatment of HIV, which we saw as the core of our mandate, turned into another issue in our relationship with the reserve health centres. In the fall of 2016, a community member tested positive for HIV in an off-reserve clinic and then returned to live back in the community. The community health nurse (CHN) was not allowed to report the positive result to the patient, and so our physician team was asked to assist during one of our visits. Giving life-changing news is something that many physicians do on a regular basis.

We broke the news. However, ongoing support and follow-up for this patient was left in the hands of the CHN. We were new to the clinic and unfamiliar with the CHN's support role, and we didn't see it as our role to offer guidance unless asked. The CHN and her nurse colleague met with the client and then moved to have a meeting with some extended family. We were not present for this meeting, but we learned that the patient left the community shortly after. He returned once to the health centre where he was seen by Stu and Susanne, but he was extremely concerned with confidentiality on the reserve and again disappeared.

Since this time, we've had occasional interactions with this client at clinics in Regina or on nursing team visits to the reserve, but we have been relatively unsuccessful in bringing him into care for his HIV condition. At the time of the writing of this chapter, he has no fixed address. He is homeless.

This story highlights some of the challenges related to HIV in Saskatchewan. First, there is limited access to HIV care and specialist support in rural and remote communities. Second, there continues to be significant stigma and a lack of understanding about the realities of HIV in rural communities, including on reserve. As a result, many individuals with HIV, as we have come to learn, have concerns about confidentiality. Whether those concerns are real or perceived is irrelevant, especially when we see the negative effects on individual health and community health.

We modified our structure and procedures, and we carried on. We were committed to the work, knowing how many patients were still showing up in the city with end-stage conditions. HIV and Hepatitis C infections were talked about as a priority at the provincial Ministry of Health, but not enough to provide funding for our clinics, at least not yet. It has to be said of Val Desjarlais that her advocacy and determination in finding federal dollars carried us through the first stages of Wellness Wheel.

AN EXPANDING CIRCLE

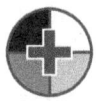

It is late on a cold, blustery December night. My phone lights up with a text from Susanne: "I'll pick you up at 8:00 a.m." I confirm with a text. I pack a lunch and lay out my clothes for the morning. It will be dark when I get up; at our latitude, the sun rises after 9:00 a.m. at this time of year. It will be a two-hour ride to the Touchwood Hills in Susanne's SUV. I am grateful for door-to-door transportation service for my work with Wellness Wheel.

A tall, willowy woman twenty years my junior, Susanne is now our project's first full-time team member and a delight to work with. Just a year after Stu Skinner hatched the idea for Wellness Wheel, Susanne began organizing our clinics on reserve, keeping the physicians informed about the dates, buying equipment, collaborating with health directors on reserve, and arranging transportation. She does everything from driving us to reserve to drawing blood to sweeping the floor.

Our conversation in the car is fun and insightful. With our coffee cups in hand, we talk about our personal lives. Susanne is planning a wedding in the spring, and we discuss dresses and flowers. As the early morning sun glistens on the snow drifting across the highway, our thoughts turn to our work. As a nurse, Susanne has had extensive experience with managing HIV. Her goal in treatment is to reduce the patient's viral load to the point where it is undetectable. With HIV, U=U; in other words, undetectable equals untransmissible.

My understanding of HIV science has been gathered in bits and pieces; the virus was identified after I graduated from medical school. The first antiviral medication for HIV was introduced in 1987, and only prolonged a patient's life for a few months. A decade later, HAART (highly active antiretroviral therapy) became the standard treatment, and now people are living longer. In fact, recent data indicates that people living with HIV, if they engage in care and take the prescribed treatment, can live as long as people who do not have HIV.[1]

Susanne starts talking about the Saskatchewan Roughriders, Regina's beloved professional football team. She tells me the story of an infamous football player recruited to Regina.

Trevis Smith was an African American player from Alabama who was with the Roughriders for seven years. During that time, he had sexual relationships with several women. It was later revealed that he failed to disclose that he was living with HIV. Eventually, one of the women found out about two other women and Smith's HIV status. She filed charges against him in 2005. The court found him guilty of not disclosing his status. He was jailed in Canada on the basis of nondisclosure, served time in a federal penitentiary, and was deported back to the US once his sentence had been completed.

People with HIV may have an undetectable viral load, where the antiretroviral treatment suppresses the HIV to such a low level that it

---

[1] Julia L. Marcus, Wendy A. Leyden, Stacey E. Alexeeff, et al., "Comparison of Overall and Comorbidity-Free Life Expectancy between Insured Adults with and without HIV Infection, 2000–2016," *JAMA Network Open* 3, no. 6 (June 15, 2020), e207954, https://doi.org/10.1001/jamanetworkopen.2020.7954.

cannot be detected on standard blood tests. People with an undetectable viral load cannot pass on the virus through sexual activity. The Public Health Act (1994) in Saskatchewan states that you must disclose your HIV status to every partner, regardless of viral load, type of activity, whether a condom or other barrier is used, or whether on treatment or not. The act has never been updated or revised to accommodate the advances in HIV care, treatment, and testing.

Our conversation in the car continues, as Susanne tells me about her experience as a public health nurse. For every hundred people with HIV in Canada, approximately seventy have contracted it from same-sex partners, twenty from heterosexual partners, and ten from sharing needles and related drug paraphernalia with people who use injection drugs. People who use drugs may come from any socio-economic background; however in Saskatchewan Indigenous people are significantly overrepresented in both the drug-using population and among those living with HIV. As she drives, Susanne fills me in on the Health Authority's contact tracing and needle exchange and distribution programs. Finding contacts is an important part of public health procedure, as we have clearly seen more recently during the COVID-19 pandemic. Pre-COVID, public health nurses like Susanne worked to track down all reported or known contacts of people living with HIV.

She often travelled to North Central Regina to knock on doors, driving an official vehicle and wearing an ID tag. Many times, people would not open the door. When they did, she would say, "Your name was given to me. You may have been in contact with someone who is HIV positive....Let's discuss a plan. You can go to the HIV clinic for free testing....Do you need a ride? Or I can test you in your own home…"

It sounded to me like a difficult job, and a risky one; a job that has prepared her to support Wellness Wheel in our work on reserves. Due to her extensive experience with Indigenous clientele in the city, she is sensitive, empathetic, and passionate about the people we serve.

We are the medicine chest. Our car is packed with red plastic crates with wheels and collapsible handles. We carry at least four large crates containing blood collection supplies, bandages, ointments, a label maker, a blood centrifuge, swabs, different coloured tubes, syringes, and basic medicines. In separate carrying cases, we tote laptops, printers, and power cords. In a doctor's bag we carry a stethoscope, an otoscope, a blood pressure cuff, and a thermometer. With all the equipment packed into the back of the vehicle, there's only room for two people—driver and passenger—in the front seats.

On this day, the health clinic is a single-storey brick structure located across from the school and down the road from the Peoples' office. We unpack the car and wheel our supplies into the building in their plastic crates. There's a waiting room with chairs. A few patients have already arrived. They are bantering among themselves. Behind a central desk sits a woman in her early twenties who directs us down the corridor. "You can have the exam room on the left," she states with a smile, as we lug in our plastic crates.

With a sense of confusion, I make my way down a corridor with multiple doors. Each office has a name plate that identifies the occupant and their title. The community health representative (CHR), the maternal and child health worker (MCH), the community health nurse (CHN), the certified diabetes educator (CDE); each has a specific role in maintaining health programs on reserve. Some are paid by the People, some by the Tribal Health Council, some by Health Canada, some by Saskatchewan Public Health. Each one answers to a different boss, with varying levels of job protection and status within their organization.

We enter the exam room that doubles as an equipment room. There are boxes of supplies sitting on shelves, a blood pressure cuff machine on the wall, and a stand-up scale for measuring body weight. There's a desk and chair in the corner, an exam table against the wall, and a three-wheeled stool. We have to make this small space work for the two of us. I take off my coat, take out a computer and lay it on the counter, pull my stethoscope from my bag, and look at the patient list. Susanne unpacks the blood-drawing equipment and sets it on the counter beside me. We look at each other and nod. We're ready to go.

The first patient, Wanda, is a fifty-year-old woman who appears underweight and frail. She walks with a wide gait from the waiting room and sits on the exam table. I roll over to the exam table on my stool. I am slightly below her, and she looks down at me.

"Hi. I'm Dr. Boan. What can I help you with?"

She tells me, through roundabout references, about her dizziness and frequent near-falls. She's bumping into things in her home, but not actually falling. She feels like she's going to fall, but then she reaches out to the wall. She's not using a cane or a walker. She can't feel her feet. And by the way, she adds, she has not been able to gain weight. As she responds to my careful questions about her symptoms, I'm puzzled. Medical teaching and experience have taught me that 80 percent of the information needed to make a diagnosis comes from the patient's story and only 20 percent comes from the physical assessment, but I'm not getting the full picture here. I need to find out more before I can proceed to the exam. Multiple things could be causing these symptoms, but I strongly suspect that she has peripheral neuropathy—a numbness in the legs or arms that results from the nerve damage caused by diabetes.

I turn to my laptop. Saskatchewan eHealth is a provincial laboratory database that allows physicians access to results from any lab and prescriptions from any pharmacy in the province. A number in the results from her most recent lab work, from over a year ago, jumps out at me—her hemoglobin A1c is high. Then I look at her medication list; she's on insulin. She hasn't mentioned that she's diabetic, despite my previous questions about her health.

I scoot back from my computer to the exam table, moving my feet to pull the three-wheeled stool closer to her.

"Your labs and medications show that you're diabetic." She looks down and nods. I interpret her downward-cast eyes as embarrassment. I need to tread gently into this territory of shame.

"Well, that's good to know. Maybe we can fix your falling," I say brightly. She raises her head, hope in her eyes, looks into my eyes, and smiles at me.

My initial suspicion is confirmed with the physical exam. She needs to improve her diabetic control in order to improve her symptoms. I recognize the difficult place that I am in. It is important to gain her trust. She did not recognize that her symptoms were related to diabetes, did not divulge her diabetes status until I found it, and looked embarrassed when I gently confirmed it with her. I cannot close this interview easily. Although I have seen some physicians confront patients with a statement like "Well, if you took better care of your diabetes, you wouldn't be falling," this is clearly not the right approach to take with Wanda.

As I delve deeper into her health problems, I discover that her dizziness always happens at the same time of day, in the afternoons. On a couple of occasions, she has taken her blood sugar, and it was low. I only have a couple of data points, since she does not take her blood sugar at home very often. At this point, I realize that she is on too much insulin in the morning, and hypoglycemia may be her problem.

With this background, her complaint about weight loss makes sense. It turns out that her cupboards are bare and her fixed budget doesn't allow extra food. She is living on income assistance and has a grandson that she cares for in her home. With the cost of heating her house on reserve and maintaining an old car for transportation, there isn't a lot left over at the end of the month. She is struggling, and I want to help her. I give her a prescription for a liquid food supplement—an item that will be covered from the Health Canada funding allocated for the health needs of Indigenous people through the Non-Insured Health Benefits program—and connect her to the Meals on Wheels program on reserve. We finish the visit with a modification of her insulin dosing and a change in one of her pills.

This first patient of my day is normally booked for twenty minutes, and we have gone over time. Susanne tells me that the waiting room is full. If each patient gives me a story that I need to untangle, we will be in the clinic later than usual. Some of the patients joke that I am working on "Indian time." Luckily, the next few patients have problems easily resolved: refills on prescriptions, yeast infection, skin infection, urinary tract infection, headache. Some take longer than others, but I don't rush. We put in a full day.

+ + +

As our visits to the Touchwood Hills reserves continued, the support system for Wellness Wheel became more formal. We attracted doctors, nurses, researchers, and administrative assistants that augmented our mission. A great early addition to our team was an Indigenous dermatologist, Dr. Rachel Asiniwasis. Rachel is of Plains Cree and Saulteaux background on her father's side, and her mother is an English immigrant. Her father is a residential school Survivor of nine years, and one of the founders of Saskatchewan's First Nations University. Her last name, Asiniwasis, translates into "Stone child" in oral Cree, and it has been passed down to her that her middle name, Netahe, means "my heart." She does have a heart for Indigenous people.

Back in Regina, we had monthly group meetings over lunch in a conference room above the Family Medicine Unit. The FMU is located in the Crossings, a renovated two-storey supermarket at Albert Street and Dewdney Avenue. This is just outside downtown Regina and at the edge of North Central, a 185-square-block area tagged as "Canada's worst neighbourhood" by *Maclean's* magazine in 2007[2] and home to many Indigenous people. The monthly meetings brought together family physicians from the FMU, physician specialists, Wellness Wheel nurses, researchers, and administrative assistants. Stu Skinner usually attended by speakerphone from his office at the Regina General Hospital. Carla Crozier, Stu's assistant, organized the agenda and chaired the meetings. She had also registered Wellness Wheel as a not-for-profit health organization under provincial regulations.

Our agenda often focused on the overlapping case load between the Touchwood Hills reserves and the city's hospitals and clinics. We talked about work standards for delivery of clinical care, sharing patient information through the electronic medical records (EMR), how to manage abnormal lab tests, and who should take the after-hours calls.

As health care providers working with Indigenous people, we spent hours discussing the protection of patient information. This is a huge concern for an Indigenous population that has sometimes been treated as an object of medical research. We wanted to keep track of our successes and failures at Wellness Wheel and share our experience with other medical teams, but we faced institutional barriers. One of these was the Personal Health Information Protection Act, which, understandably, restricts the disclosure of individual health data. The other was the principles listed in the ownership, control, access, and possession system. More commonly known by its registered trademark acronym, OCAP is administered by a non-profit organization called the First Nations Information Governance Centre. It asserts that First Nations have control over data collection processes in their communities, and they own and control how this information can be

---

2   Jonathon Gatehouse, "Ten years later, we ask again: What's wrong in Regina?" *Maclean's*, January 23, 2017, https://macleans.ca/news/canada/ten-years-later-we-ask-again-whats-wrong-in-regina/.

used.³ In other words, we needed to negotiate with each band council around any sharing of any insights gained from our work.

The physician members of the team all had full-time jobs. We took vacation days or cancelled private-practice office days in order to travel to reserve. Val Desjarlais, the Touchwood Agency Tribal Council's health manager, had now secured funding from her Government of Canada contacts to cover a daily stipend for family doctors. I was still excluded, on the assumption that my specialist's billing rate at the reserve clinics would be enough compensation. Each driver submitted their mileage to Val and was reimbursed; each family physician submitted an invoice to Val after a clinic day on reserve and was paid as a contractor. None of these funds flowed through Wellness Wheel.

However, the cost of running the on-reserve clinics required other supports such as nursing, phone calls, computers, and office space for support staff. Carla Crozier managed the Wellness Wheel accounts while Susanne and Stu looked for creative ways to use limited funds from the federal and provincial governments to support nursing services. As the team's credibility grew, so did our ability to beg or borrow resources from various health agencies. We borrowed two clinical researchers, Adam and Mamata, on part-time loan from the Saskatchewan Health Authority (SHA). Dr. Stephanie Konrad, an epidemiologist, joined us from Health Canada; a nurse named Maria was funded from federal Hepatitis C Research Initiative funds; and the University of Regina provided a short-term IT support person, a health information management student who required a work-study semester. As Carla told me: "Overall, the reason for our success was a 'let's just do it' attitude. If we had taken the time to fully integrate Wellness Wheel with the SHA bureaucracy, we would still be in planning meetings. The

---

3   "The First Nations Principles of OCAP®," First Nations Information Governance Centre, https://fnigc.ca/.

'let's just do it' attitude provided us with the flexibility we needed to provide care on reserve."

Even so, each physician continued to work at other jobs—practising family medicine in the Regina Family Medicine Unit, teaching medical students, working at the hospital, seeing private patients in private offices. Dr. Rosie Courtney, for example, worked in the hospital ER full-time and went to clinics on reserve once per month. My participation was limited by my commitment to the Regina General, which required me to work at least seven days per month as a consulting specialist in Internal Medicine. Other doctors had more extensive hospital commitments, up to a minimum of fifteen days per month. Our schedules were and are haphazard, depending on the prevalence of various health conditions across the province and the health of our individual patients. One step towards a more orderly process came at the request of TATC Health Director Val Desjarlais; she asked Susanne to assign each family doctor to an individual reserve, with a scheduled visit at least once a month. Specialists would go to the different reserves on a rotating basis, except where there was an urgent need.

As I spent more time on reserve, I was able to improve the *continuity of care*—somewhat of a buzzword in the medical community—for people who travelled back and forth between the reserve and the city. I often met patients from the Touchwood Hills in my hospital rounds in Regina and was able to say, "I'll see you on my next visit to your community"; travelling to the reserve for a clinic day, I would meet with patients who had been discharged from hospital and wanted follow-up.

I also met with new patients, more each year, who came because they had heard about us by word of mouth. In between visits, we maintained an on-call team roster to respond to emergencies, communicating alerts through an online patient database with a messaging feature.

My connection with the hospital and specialists in the hospital also worked the other way. If I saw a patient on reserve that needed care quickly but non-emergently, I would ask them to come into the city and meet me at the hospital. In many cases, Susanne would text me when the patient was leaving reserve. Back in Regina, when a patient arrived at the triage desk of the ER, they could say, "I'm here to meet Dr. Boan." The ER nurse would call me; I would leave the medical ward and go downstairs and greet them. I would inform the ER physician and then arrange a bed placement number so the patient could be admitted and moved upstairs, allowing their treatment to begin immediately. I'm happy to compare this procedure with the fast-tracking that routinely happens with more privileged patients whose need for care is established. I do not feel any guilt for making the system work in the way it is designed to work.

The Wellness Wheel budget was growing, built with bits and pieces scrounged from various government programs. However, our budget was tiny compared to the total amount of money spent on Indigenous health services in Saskatchewan. In fact, as Waldram, Herring, and Young state in their book *Aboriginal Health in Canada*,[4] nobody knows how much money is spent in the name of Indigenous health services. With all the agencies, programs, institutes, nations, societies, consortiums, and volunteer teams, there is no bottom line and no road map to tell the general public who is paying for what.

Speculating on the cost of Indigenous health care leads us into a world of mystery. When a patient is admitted to the hospital, the Saskatchewan Health plan pays the costs. Fine. But if the patient has a status card, the cost can then be billed from Saskatchewan to the Government of Canada. Or part of the cost. The provincial public servant who asks for a payment from Ottawa doesn't really know the cost

---

4   James B. Waldram, D. Ann Herring, and T. Kue Young, *Aboriginal Health in Canada: Historical, Cultural and Epidemiological Perspectives* (Toronto: University of Toronto Press, 2007).

of the patient's hospital stay. And then, through different channels, Ottawa transfers funds to Saskatchewan from its general revenues to cover provincial costs for health care and is also making special payments to the provinces through Indigenous Services Canada to support First Nations health. All to support a system that, in the end, is producing inferior health outcomes for Indigenous people.

Jurisdiction is a triggering word for all people living on reserve. Who has jurisdiction? Leadership in Indigenous communities has been referred from Ottawa to the provincial capital in Regina, and then back to Ottawa. Wellness Wheel deals with jurisdictional disputes daily—all it takes is a walk down a corridor in one of the Indigenous community's health clinics.

When I first arrived on reserve, I assumed that the health clinic was separated from the community in the same way a clinic in the city is separated from the community. When you see a patient in an urban clinic, the average physician looks at the medical problem and treats the medical problem. The social determinants of health still don't usually form a primary part of the diagnosis, with possible exceptions such as HIV, Hep C, alcoholism, domestic abuse, and rape. Even in those cases, the police, public health, psychiatry, or social workers are called in an attempt to solve the problem. Most of the time in the city, the physician treats the disease—high blood pressure, diabetes, or cancer screening.

Over time I learned that the health clinic on reserve is a different entity. It embodies (in a very imperfect way) everything in a very small community—suicide prevention, mental health support, and responses to residential school trauma, poverty, homelessness, affordable housing, transportation, and drug addiction.

Health Canada, with its rules of engagement and mandatory structures, tries to put each Indigenous community into the same neat box. For lack of other options, and to keep the money flowing, Indigenous organizations try to comply with the funding rules. Yet, the community is a living organism that struggles to connect the past to the present through generations of hereditary knowledge and more recent experience. It is not a neat box. Health Canada and all the other institutions need to learn two-eyed seeing and engage their community partners. With Wellness Wheel, we have attempted to overcome the biases inherent in a bureaucratic system that focuses on putting up walls. We are on a mission to understand how a community can take control of its own health.

THE MISSION STATEMENT FOR WELLNESS WHEEL

- *Community Driven*: Indigenous people's self-determination is the foundation of our values. Everything we do is focused on meeting the needs of Indigenous individuals, families, and communities, based upon their input. We support community empowerment to ensure Wellness Wheel is Indigenous led and locally adapted to meet specific needs.

- *Culturally Based*: Indigenous ways of knowing, doing, and being inform and guide our relationships, methods, and practices. We provide accessible services in a safe, supportive environment for our clients.

- *Relationship Focused*: We work to establish trusted and respected relationships with Indigenous individuals, families, and communities by being transparent as our "real selves" so our clients can be their "real selves." There is no hierarchy in our relationships and we treat every person with respect and unconditional positive regard.

- *Strengths Based Approach*: While we do not ignore the realities of disease, we focus on a strengths based health promotion approach that facilitates wellness by building on the pathways of strength and resilience. We take a compassionate, empathetic, and trauma-informed approach to ensure our clients feel safe and protected.

- *Streamlined & Patient Centered Care*: We are committed to providing outcome based care that meets the needs of an individual in a friendly and safe environment. Our multi-disciplinary team involving primary care and specialists prides itself on regular communication, within the team and to the patient, to facilitate care that minimizes the time for diagnostic tests, treatment, and the need for travel.

- *Local & Action Oriented*: Community development, ownership, and capacity building are significant factors that are present at all service levels (i.e., design, delivery, implementation, and evaluation) when enhancing wellness in First Nations communities. Sustainable and effective community development initiatives involve community capacity building with a strong focus on inherent strengths within First Nations communities.

- *Ethical & Responsible*: We are committed to maintaining privacy and confidentiality at all times and conducting ethical research on improving Indigenous health outcomes and outreach in compliance with the First Nations principles of OCAP® (Ownership, Control, Access, and Possession).[5]

---

5   *Wellness Wheel Medical Clinic: Strategic Direction Overview*, unpublished paper, 2019.

RED DRESS DAY

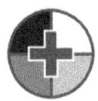

Patricia is lying in a private room in the hospital with her hair done and makeup on. I am standing by her bedside, fashionably dressed in a pencil skirt and blouse. My thin blonde hair is cut to my shoulders; my makeup is understated. As a woman in a male-dominated field, I am careful to dress conservatively. Both Patricia and I have been trained in the world of patriarchy. We are two women that have learned to manoeuvre in a man's world, each of us with a different story of patriarchy.

While her smile lights up the room, her heart is infected for the second time. She has fevers and chest pain. The chart says she was treated a year ago for a bacterial infection of the tricuspid heart valve, a condition she picked up from using a dirty needle while injecting drugs.[1]

At that time, our infectious disease service treated her with intravenous antibiotics. She completed a six-week course of treatment in hospital and went home. The experience scared her, and she vowed never

---

1   Infections such as these due to drug use are being seen with increasing frequency, not only among Indigenous people. Ishba M. Syed, Bobby Yanagawa, Suganthiny Jeyaganth, Subodh Verma, and Asim N. Cheema, "Injection Drug Use Endocarditis: An Inner-City Hospital Experience," *CJC Open* 3, no. 7 (March 9, 2021): 896–903, https://doi.org/10.1016/j.cjco.2021.02.015.

to do drugs again. She stayed clean for a year. Recently, she relapsed and came to the ER for help. She was admitted to the medical ward last night and assigned to my care.

She asks first for something to help with her chest pain. Before determining how much narcotic medicine I should order for her, I need to know her usual dose. If her body is used to big doses of narcotics, the mini doses that we usually prescribe for opioid-naive patients will not be enough. After she tells me how much Dilaudid—a prescription pain killer often sold on the street—she has been regularly taking, I write an order for a whopping dose of scheduled narcotics.

Why Patricia is having chest pain, and what causes chest pain in patients with infected valves, requires a brief medical explanation. The heart has four chambers divided into two sides, left and right. The left heart, made up of the left atrium and left ventricle, pumps oxygenated blood to the body, perfusing all the organs, including the brain and kidneys, as well as the limbs. The blood then flows back to the right heart through the veins. The right heart (the right atrium and right ventricle) takes the "blue" or used-up blood and pumps it into the lungs, filling it with oxygen.

The valve separating the right ventricle from the right atrium is called the tricuspid valve. When a person injects drugs into their veins, the injected drug mixes with the blue blood and goes to the right heart. The tricuspid valve is bathed with any bacteria entering the bloodstream from a dirty needle. Some of the bacteria stick to the valve and begin to replicate, forming a vegetative cover. A heart valve that has been previously damaged is at higher risk for reinfection.

Small pieces of the vegetation sometimes break off from the valve and go to the lungs. These showers of bacteria are called septic emboli. They get stuck in the lung tissue and begin to grow. Bacterial infection in the lungs, similar to pneumonia, can cause chest pain, a common complaint among people who use drugs.

Those who use drugs, irrespective of ethnicity, are high utilizers of the health care system. A study of almost six hundred people in Vancouver in the late 1990s showed that people who use drugs, from all backgrounds, visited the Emergency Room three times per year on average, with 20 percent going to the Emergency Room more than ten times per year.[2] We have noticed similar trends in Regina, although we have not collected the data to document the use of the ER by people who use drugs. But we are aware that the Emergency Rooms are overflowing. Without a doubt, the crisis in ER wait times is linked to limited access to medical care in the outpatient setting.

In many cases, people who use drugs arrive with diseases that have been untreated and have progressed to the point where they need a stay in hospital to recover. Another study that looked at urban poverty in Canada and hospital admission rates in the early 1990s found that more people from poor neighbourhoods are admitted to hospital.[3] The commonest causes for admission to hospital for people that use drugs are pneumonia and infections, with almost 60 percent of the cases requiring frequent admissions. In my experience at the Regina General Hospital, Indigenous people with drug-related infections tend to occupy more than half the private rooms (isolation rooms), which are in short supply. Care for these patients requires gowning and special sanitary protocols.[4] Members of the hospital team estimate that

---

2 A. Palepu, M.W. Tyndall, H. Leon, J. Muller, M.V. O'Shaughnessy, M.T. Schechter, and A.H. Anis, "Hospital Utilization and Costs in a Cohort of Injection Drug Users," *Canadian Medical Association Journal* 165, no. 4 (August 21, 2001): 415–420, https://pubmed.ncbi.nlm.nih.gov/11531049/.

3 R.H. Glazier, E.M. Badley, J.E. Gilbert, and L. Rothman, "The Nature of Increased Hospital Use in Poor Neighbourhoods: Findings from a Canadian Inner City," *The Canadian Journal of Public Health* 91, no. 4 (July–August 2000): 268–273, https://doi.org/10.1007/BF03404286.

4 Charles E. Cherubin and Joseph D. Sapira, "The Medical Complications of Drug Addiction and the Medical Assessment of the Intravenous Drug User: 25 Years...

for each episode of bacterial heart and lung infection, the cost to the taxpayer is approximately $50,000.[5]

If governments and health care administrators ever decide to address the underlying causes of drug addiction, I believe that it will reduce our health care costs as well as the level of human suffering related to drug use and related illness. I have had almost daily contact with patients who sit in front of me, trapped in emotional turmoil, wanting to escape from drugs and have a life free of them. Unfortunately, I'm unable to provide either the social supports—the housing security, for example—or the therapeutic supports that are needed to give drug users a real chance at a new life. And in Saskatchewan, some of the people who control the health care budgets take the view that drug users are bad, lazy, untrustworthy people who, with their drug use, have forfeited any right to support.

Intravenous drug use is associated with increased risk of HIV and Hepatitis C. Fortunately, Patricia's tests for these conditions came back negative, but her blood cultures are positive for *staphylococcus* bacteria. As we meet for the first time, I don't know what has caused Patricia to relapse into her drug habit. For the moment, it doesn't matter. I don't ask her about it. She doesn't need my judgments. She doesn't need me to tell her she made a mistake. She needs medical care. However, her second admission to hospital for an infected heart valve means another long stay and another course of IV antibiotics.

But she begins to volunteer her story without my prompting. She wants to get better because she has three kids, and she wants to see

---

...Later," *Annals of Internal Medicine* 119 (November 15, 1993): 1017–1028, https://doi.org/10.7326/0003-4819-119-10-199311150-00009.

[5] Aaron T. Fleischauer, Laura Ruhl, Sarah Rhea, and Erin Barnes, "Hospitalizations for Endocarditis and Associated Health Care Costs Among Persons with Diagnosed Drug Dependence — North Carolina, 2010-2015," *MMWR* and *Morbidity and Mortality Weekly Rep* 66, no. 22 (June 9, 2017): 569–573, http://dx.doi.org/10.15585/mmwr.mm6622a1.

them. Unfortunately, her ex-husband, whom she describes as abusive, has custody. I have fought my own bruising rounds with the child custody system, and I still don't really understand how it is supposed to work. In my case, it wasn't the government's social workers who were trying to take my child away from me; it was a bitter ex-husband advocating for full custody. Even as a privileged white doctor, I was forced into years of court battles so I could maintain access to my child. I can only imagine the barriers that Patricia has faced; her world is so far removed from mine. It's clear she has come out on the short end.

Since her staph infection creates an infection risk for everyone around her, she has been given a private room. She is settled in comfortably with her cosmetics carefully laid out on her bedside table. She tells me that she has accepted her present fate and will get back to fighting for her children when she gets out of the hospital. We both know that it will be an uphill battle with Child and Family Services. In the meantime, she plans to lie back and enjoy the relative quiet of the hospital.

Patricia then says she sometimes works on the street. She says she could earn as much as $8,000 per month if she wanted to, having sex with men in downtown hotel rooms. This would be more than enough money to support her kids. "So why are the child protection workers giving me a hard time?" she asks. I am moved by her resilience to survive in a patriarchal world.

Through meeting Patricia, I am learning about the struggles of women who are subjugated by men, even endangered by them in order to survive. While I operate in a male-dominated career, I have no idea of the strength it takes to overcome the barriers that she is faced with. As her doctor, I cannot provide a solution to these problems. I want to be able to offer the love and support she needs to take on the obstacles, but my role is limited. I wonder how my male colleagues see these sorts of situations. Do they feel helpless, too?

The number of women entering medical school has increased over time, but female physicians experience misogyny on a daily basis. In the minds of many hospitalized patients, every woman on staff is a nurse and every man is a doctor, and I am regularly summoned as "sweetie" by hospitalized patients to bring a blanket or a urinal to pee into. My male physician colleagues are accustomed to working with women, but the medical power structure continues to be male dominated. On average, women physicians earn less than men with equal training for equal work. A woman like myself who is tall and self-confident is often labeled a "dragon lady"; if I were a man, I would more likely be described as powerful and successful. Every female professional in the system—doctor, nurse, pharmacist, administrator—learns to manoeuvre in order to survive. I have watched female colleagues display coquettish behavior in a room full of male colleagues, angling to get what they want by flirting subtly and playing to the fragile egos of some men. As they snuggle up to the men at work or on social occasions, I see that they often succeed. Suddenly, their research project is funded, or the hospital program that was threatened is back on track. They play the game. In my conversation with Patricia, I get the message that she understands the system of male power. She doesn't need to spell out the details about how she operates. The difference is I have a ticket in the door to power because I'm white and privileged. I don't have to sell my body to be invited into the room.

Many of my colleagues in health care take the view that prostitution among Indigenous women is the result of white dominance and the loss of traditional culture. This is a valid perspective, although I don't buy the idea that life on Turtle Island was pure and simple in pre-contact times (the oral histories provide evidence of slavery, warfare, and family dysfunction). In any case, when Europeans first began to explore the continent and harvest furs for shipment to Europe, they found Indigenous women to be strong and capable. Historian Sylvia Van

Kirk's account, *Many Tender Ties—Women in Fur-Trade Society, 1670–1870*, lists the skills that the Indigenous woman brought to the voyageur expedition: cooking, gathering food, dressing skins, drying meat, making a fire, carrying children, paddling a canoe. She knew how to gather gum for mending canoes. She could make snowshoes, moccasins, and leather garments. She gathered berries, dried the meat, and packed pemmican. She often spoke many languages, and she understood the land, acting as guide and negotiator. She was essential to the white fur trader's survival, although the role of women was never mentioned in our 1960s schoolrooms.

As the fur trade became more organized, towards 1800, corporate headquarters decreed that Indigenous partners or helpers (and the children that white employees had fathered) could no longer live within the walls of the fort or trading post. There are reports that, as a result, the wives and partners sometimes camped nearby. Over time, some tribes began to sell the favours of their women if they had nothing else to trade. The addition of alcohol addiction to this picture had a further demoralizing effect.[6] As logging camps and prostitution increased in popularity, survival sex was the way out of a demoralizing life on reserve.

Métis author, filmmaker, and Elder Maria Campbell's evocative autobiography, published in 1973, was a testimony to the risks faced by women of Indigenous ancestry.[7] In her story, Campbell leaves her home in Saskatchewan for the streets of Vancouver. Through the course of her heart-wrenching narrative about her interaction with illicit drugs and prostitution—products of a lifetime of alienation and low self-esteem—she throws off the blanket of shame.

---

6   Sylvia Van Kirk, *Many Tender Ties: Women in Fur-Trade Society, 1670–1870* (Norman, Oklahoma: University of Oklahoma Press, 1980).

7   Maria Campbell, *Halfbreed* (Lincoln, Nebraska: University of Nebraska Press, 1973).

Whatever the process, the association between Indigenous women and prostitution became anchored in the minds of white men, and it continues to put women in danger. Around the time that I met Patricia in hospital, an Indigenous woman was found dead at the bottom of a laundry chute in one of Regina's downtown hotels, having fallen ten storeys to her death. The inquest was inconclusive, and the perpetrators, if any, simply walked away.

In another hospital room on the same floor where Patricia is staying, I treat a male patient with gallstones. He tells me that he's a ringleader in the prostitution scene in Regina. Maybe because he trusts me, or regards me as naive, he confides in me. He speaks about the case of the woman and the laundry chute, and about the judges, lawyers, politicians, and businessmen who come to that hotel. Names that I recognize—powerful men with wives, families, and honourable social positions. I thank him for his candor, but I am disgusted by this description of Regina's social underbelly, particularly as a woman who deals with misogyny on a daily basis. Patricia, in a different part of the hospital, is dealing with an infected heart valve that resulted from the trading of sex for money.

Any Indigenous woman who has travelled along a public highway in Canada over the past hundred years has run the risk of being assaulted or murdered. I remember the outrage that I felt in 2003 when Robert Pickton was being prosecuted as a serial killer of sex workers from Vancouver's Downtown Eastside. It was horrifying front-page news. As early as 2014, the RCMP report "Missing and Murdered Aboriginal Women: A National Operational Overview"[8]

---

8   RCMP's 2014 report *Missing and Murdered Aboriginal Women: A National Operational Overview* had in its records 225 open and unsolved cases of missing or murdered Indigenous women dating back to 1980, including 105 who had been missing for more than thirty days and 120 unsolved homicides. https://...

was criticized as underestimating the true numbers.[9,10] Then Tina Lafontaine's body was discovered in the Red River near Winnipeg. A fifteen-year-old, wrapped in a blanket and weighed down with rocks, Tina had been murdered by a white man. By 2016, a national inquiry was funded by the Government of Canada to explore the systemic causes behind the violence that plagued Indigenous women. Its report recognized racism, poverty, addiction, sexual exploitation, the over-representation of Indigenous children in the child welfare system, inadequate on-reserve housing, inadequate education opportunities, insufficient public transit, and domestic violence.[11] Every year on May 5, I wear a red dress to work to remember these victims of colonization and think of the part that Patricia played in introducing me to the systems of power that control women's bodies. The symbolism of the red dresses was originated by Métis artist Jaime Black in 2010. In her REDress Project exhibit, Black displayed over one hundred red dresses around the University of Winnipeg campus to raise awareness. It caught on, and today red dresses are used across Canada and the United States as a representation of the Indigenous

---

...www.rcmp-grc.gc.ca/en/missing-and-murdered-aboriginal-women-national-operational-overview.

9 In the Native Women's Association of Canada's 2010 "Missing and Murdered Aboriginal Women and Girls in Saskatchewan" fact sheet analysis of 582 cases of disappearance or murder in Saskatchewan, more than 40 percent of the Indigenous women who were murdered died on roadways or in open areas; 36 percent who were murdered died at the hands of strangers, and the relationship between victim and killer is unknown in a further 28 percent of cases.

10 Indigenous women are roughly seven times more likely to be slain by a serial killer than non-Indigenous women. Kathryn Blaze Baum and Matthew McClearn, "Prime Target: How Serial Killers Prey on Indigenous Women," *Globe and Mail*, November 22, 2015, https://www.theglobeandmail.com/news/national/prime-targets-serial-killers-and-indigenous-women/article27435090/.

11 *Reclaiming Power and Place: The Final Report of the National Inquiry into Missing and Murdered Indigenous Women and Girls*. Canada, 2019. Web archive. https://www.loc.gov/item/lcwaN0028038/.

women and girls lost to violent crime and as a call for action to prevent future violence.[12]

I never see Patricia again after she is discharged from hospital. I don't know if she regained custody of her children. I don't know if she was able to shake off the lure of income supplementation that comes from sex work. I do know that she had the strength to adjust to changing circumstances. I do know, with her intelligence and beauty, that she is (or was) a Survivor.

✢ ✢ ✢

My encounter with Patricia took place during the time when the Wellness Wheel project was in its formative stages. Stu Skinner and our growing team had chosen to focus on the rural Indigenous communities as a way of making measurable gains among people who had limited access to health care.

Unfortunately, Wellness Wheel did not have the resources to open up a second location in the inner city. I would like to offer continuity of care through Wellness Wheel to women who work on the street. Patricia had resilience, but she also had a host of factors working against her. Women in Patricia's circumstances are often viewed, by authorities, social workers, health care professionals, and the white population generally, as second-class citizens. "Native girl syndrome" is an old-fashioned sociological phrase that highlights this bias; it can be used in a casual, quasi-professional way to describe any behaviour among Indigenous women disapproved of by the dominant society. The phrase has its silent equivalents in the look from the ER nurses when someone like Patricia comes into the waiting room and the unease among the

---

12 "About the REDress Project," Indigenous Foundations, First Nations & Indigenous Studies at the University of British Columbia, https://indigenousfoundations.arts.ubc.ca/about_the_redress_project/.

porters who wheel the patients up to their rooms. I hear it in the voice of the exasperated head nurse who complains that someone has signed herself out of hospital AMA (against medical advice). Again.

For the subset of Indigenous women who are working in the sex trade the risks are very high. In theory it is a lucrative business, but it is a business linked with perils. It is often associated with drug addiction and sexually transmitted infections (STI), which is linked in turn to chronic illness and early death. I ponder: What is my role in treating these women? How does racial stigma, feminization of poverty, and the danger of being labeled as an unfit mother interact with my role as a physician? As for those who are not inclined to delve further into issues of colonization or racism, we might look instead at the cost of continued poor health among Indigenous people—reframing the argument that addressing these issues has financial implications as well as social ones.

MICHAEL'S TEARS

There is a mysterious rhythm to hospital admissions. Some days are quiet, with a steady but modest flow of people into the Emergency Room. At other times the place is a circus, with the waiting room full, people sleeping on benches by the swinging entrance door, people in wheelchairs waiting to be assessed, and ambulances pulling up and rolling patients on gurneys into hallways. Some doctors and nurses speculate that it has something to do with the phase of the moon, but I know of no clear explanation for everyone getting sick on the same day. And when people come in to the ER, they tend to remain in the ER, even after they have been officially admitted for treatment. The ER functions as a holding area because Regina General, like many hospitals across Canada, is always full.

Some days and nights are so busy that no one has time to talk; we just move from one patient to the next. Quick thinking, astute diagnoses, recognizing what's dangerous, calling the appropriate subspecialists, writing the correct management orders. No time to relax. No time to pee. No time for a glass of water. The goal of the Emergency team is to complete a quick assessment and move the patient to a bed upstairs or out the door, as appropriate. As a senior physician on the Internal Medicine wards, I am obliged to accept who the ER sends us—the sick patients who have no other place to go. If they don't qualify for surgery, pediatrics, obstetrics, or psychiatry, then Internal Medicine is their new home.

When it gets busy in the ER, there is a palpable change in energy. The staff work together like a well-oiled machine: triage nurse takes history, patient moves into a bed, nurse takes vitals, ER physician does history and physical, decision for admission is made. Blood is drawn for preliminary lab tests. Unit clerk is informed of the need to consult with Internal Medicine. On most days, my pager does not go off, since I am already at the centre of the action, and I have already seen a series of very sick patients—acute congestive heart failure, acute exacerbation of COPD, sepsis, confusion, liver failure.

At 8:00 p.m., Debbie, the unit clerk, taps me on the shoulder. "Dr. Boan, there's a consult for you in room eight." I am standing outside room seven, writing orders for a very old woman from a care home who is struggling to understand where she is. After ten minutes of paperwork she is taken care of for the night, and I step towards room eight. When I finish with this one, there is someone waiting in bed nine. I don't have much time.

Room eight is at the back of the ER. Outside the room there is a counter at waist height where the paperwork lies. The heading on the ER consult sheet reads "pre-op consult." I look at the assessment sheet from the primary nurse. This patient has rated the pain in his body at 9 out of a possible 10.

- *Subjective data*: 11:24 a.m.—Patient brought by ambulance from provincial jail. Patient stated while standing up to transfer from bed to wheelchair, right leg gave out on him and he fell to right side. Unable to ambulate immediately and assisted to bed by nursing staff at jail. Patient complaining of pain to right hip radiating to right side back, down to right thigh and right lower leg. No numbness or tingling sensation. Pain at present 9/10. Awaiting right hip repair by orthopedic surgeon. PHx: right hip chronic pain, left knee and thigh pain.

- *Temp*: 37.2°C
- *Heart rate*: 78
- *BP systolic*: 115
- *BP diastolic*: 66
- *O₂ saturation*: 98%
- *Additional information*: No deformity noted or reported by patient. X-ray of right hip shows greater trochanteric fracture.

I step through a door into a holding and dressing area with a chair and a small sink. At ninety degrees to my left is another door; and beyond that a second door; and, finally, room eight. *Unable to ambulate immediately and assisted to bed by nursing staff at jail.* There are two correctional officers—jail guards—seated on chairs on either side of the bed. I disregard them. I am in a hurry, and their story is not important to me.

The patient, Michael, has strong facial features that remind me of the paintings of Turtle Island people by the frontier artists from the 1800s, George Catlin[1] or Paul Kane.[2]

He is lying on his back, an IV running into his left arm. I move closer to the bedside and introduce myself. He avoids eye contact and answers my questions in a strong voice. I have learned through my

---

[1] George Catlin was an American who painted portraits of American Plains Indians from 1830 to 1836.
[2] Paul Kane, an itinerant portrait painter from Toronto, was commissioned by Sir George Simpson of the Hudson's Bay Company to document Indigenous life in Canada. He published *Wanderings of an Artist among the Indians of North America* in 1859.

training to use open-ended questions, to allow patients the freedom to elaborate. But Michael does not move into the space I allow when I invite him to tell me more about his health. Despite this, I intuitively feel personal power emanating from him. He is in pain, but he endures it with stoic grace.

The term *Noble Indian* comes into my mind, partly unwelcome, with its clutch of associations both with Indigenous activists I met in my youth and with television Indians from my childhood.[3] It is a term that is potentially insulting and politically charged. Thomas King lampoons the archetype in his book *The Inconvenient Indian*. "Dead Indians are dignified, noble, silent, suitably garbed. And dead. Live Indians are invisible, unruly, disappointing. And breathing."[4] For me, the ideal of Indigenous nobility is deeply rooted. As a university student in early 1970s Regina, I became a supporter of the revival of Indigenous spirituality and empowerment. In the era of anti–Vietnam War demonstrations, middle-class suburban youth on the Canadian prairies paid close attention to the sudden rise of a militant Indigenous leadership that did not recognize a Canadian-American border. We carried Dee Brown's *Bury My Heart at Wounded Knee* as a bible for the cause. Vine DeLoria Jr.'s book *Custer Died for Your Sins* became a bestseller and promoted the view of the Indian as wise and strong. His account as well as the writings of various popular anthropologists influenced my thinking about the Indigenous keepers of the land that I inhabited. As nomads following the buffalo on the prairies, the anthropologists wrote, people had little respect for personal possessions. They could only own as much as they could carry easily. There was no incentive to accumulate

---

3   Tonto from *The Lone Ranger*, for example, or Joe Two Rivers from Canada's own *Forest Rangers*—characters who were sometimes portrayed by First Nations actors, and sometimes not.
4   Thomas King, *The Inconvenient Indian: A Curious Account of Native People in North America* (Toronto: Anchor Canada, 2013), 66.

material goods. Their dependence on each other and the land was more important. Wealth was defined by personal relationships.

With his dignity and apparent self-awareness, Michael reminds me of the Elders I have met in the sickrooms and hallways of this hospital—people who have somehow, against the odds, maintained a spiritual view of life and have not been overrun by the dominant settler community. They are often visiting a loved one who is hospitalized and sit for hours at the bedside. They speak with me about their own experience, weaving the elements of intuition, spirit, experience, and groundedness in a specific place, often mentioning the Creator or the power of nature. The fragments of information they share with me help me understand their loved one's connection to a larger external world. With time and repeated exposure to a holistic circular approach, I am thankful that the Elders have allowed this knowledge to be shared with me.[5] The consistent message that I have received from these oral teachings is that all I can know is my own experience. And Michael expands my personal experience of the tension between the Noble Indian and servitude.

Have Turtle Island's people submitted to servitude? In some ways, yes—servitude to external conditions over which they have no control. The stories blend. Visit the ER in any Canadian prairie city: knife wounds, pneumonia, hypoxia, fevers, joint pain, chest pain, inability to walk. Admitted to the medical floor for treatment. Leaving their medical room to go down to the smoking area. Coming back with drugs. Nurses finding needles and spoons under the pillow. Confronted and accused of drug use in the hospital. Denial and lying. Anger and despair.

---

5   As settlers, we assume that we are promoting a post-colonial perspective when we use decolonizing language. I have learned that this is not the whole truth. The tension between domination and servitude underlies all settler-Indigenous interactions like a photo that has been airbrushed.

Leaving the hospital against medical advice. Reappearing days later with worse symptoms. Readmitted to the medical floor. The cycle goes on, and I am part of it.

Servitude to low paying jobs, poor education, inadequate housing. Dependence on government programs. In my mind, the "Noble Indian" is captive now. As Mi'kmaq lawyer, professor, and activist Pam Palmater stated at the Woodrow Lloyd annual lecture in 2018, "Prisons are the new residential schools, with First Nations making up 25 percent of the male prison population and 36 percent of the female prison population. Native women are 7 times more likely to be sexually abused compared to whites. There is a link between foster care and human sex trafficking. The system makes us criminals, for example the rules on hunting and trapping makes us sneak around the bush. If we defend our right to the land, we are criminals."[6]

And so, through some chain of events, Michael has landed in jail. He does not fit the image or carry the menacing air of a convicted offender. With his long braid, he appears serene and non-violent, even with his left ankle shackled to the metal bar of the hospital bed. The nature of his crime is unimportant to me. It is his medical story that concerns me. It doesn't make sense—*treated for right hip abscess two months ago*—since he now has pus coming out a tiny tunnel from his hip joint to the skin in his right hip region. Most patients with a hip fracture—the diagnosis on his medical chart—are frail and elderly or have had trauma like a skiing or car accident. I am puzzled as to why a strong forty-eight-year-old man has a broken hip. He doesn't want to tell me everything. I don't push. I put in a request for his previous medical records from another province to see if I can piece together the mystery, knowing that the information may take days to arrive.

---

6   "2018 Woodrow Lloyd Lecture," YouTube.

I order an MRI and wait for the result. Several hours later, the image shows that Michael's right hip has an abscess around the right hip bone; the abscess has infected the top of the femur bone and made the bone structure decay. It was a perfect set-up for a fracture; the weakened bone could not hold his weight when he tried to stand. I pick up the phone and call the orthopedic surgeon to let him know the MRI findings. The decision about which procedure to perform is in the surgeon's wheelhouse, not mine. The surgeon is between cases and sitting in the doctors lounge, where he pulls up the MRI images on the hospital computer. A straightforward surgical repair of the hip is no longer an option. He says, "I'll take this guy into the OR and resect his femoral head to clean out the infection." My heart sinks. The surgery will result in one leg shortening, and Michael will likely limp for the rest of his life.

We find a room for Michael in the orthopedic ward. A porter will roll him up to the fifth floor, with the two correctional officers following the bed on wheels. I see the little procession leave the ER out of the corner of my eye. By midnight I have finished admitting another two patients to the hospital. I pick up a plastic cup near the water cooler; I have been so busy, I have forgotten to eat or drink. The water cooler's hum masks the conversations among doctors and nurses, patients and families. Before I go home, I decide that I should tell Michael the plan for his surgery. But first I need to find him.

Outside the Emergency area, the hospital at night is a different place than during the day. The lights are low; patients are sleeping. The daytime hospital staff—social workers, pharmacists, food services workers pushing carts, unit clerks—are absent. It has an eerie, almost haunted feel. I walk to the centre of the orthopedic ward where the nurses are drinking coffee. They look at me strangely; I have interrupted their break with my unexpected presence. I ask about Michael, who came up from the ER earlier in the evening. After offering me a coffee that I politely refuse, they tell me he is in a private room down the hall.

There are two guards sitting outside room ten, not the same guards that accompanied Michael to the hospital. They are playing cards. I suggest, half-jokingly, that they don't need to be here since the patient can't walk and his good leg is shackled to the hospital bed. He is not going to escape. They understand, but rules are rules. They are doing their job. I am doing mine.

I enter his room after I dress in gown and gloves. Michael has been placed in isolation by Infection Control. I close the door. I don't want the guards to hear the conversation. Gossip can be evil, and I don't trust that what I share with Michael will be kept confidential. He is lying flat. The window faces northwest, looks over the hospital parking lot—towards the downtown towers, and beyond that to the coulee-riven plains of the upper Qu'Appelle River Valley. The sun has set hours ago. It is winter solstice, the longest night of the year.

"How's the pain?"

"They're giving me IV painkillers. It's okay."

"I'm here to give you the results of the MRI. It shows an abscess in the bone of the hip. You'll be going to the operating room. The surgeon will clean out the infection in your hip. I'm afraid the top of your leg bone will have to be removed."

He is stoic. He says nothing. I wait.

Tears begin falling down his face, running across his ears. No sobbing, just silent tears. He says nothing.

"I am sorry," I say. Pause, more tears are falling.

"The orthopedic surgeon will talk more with you about the procedure. We'll start antibiotics and get rid of the infection in your hip."

I sit by the side of his bed, silent for a long time. I am tired and don't want to move. I don't want to leave this man alone with this terrible news. I stay to bear witness to the tears, not tears of physical pain but tears that come from years of struggle with an unfair system. I sense that his life has not been easy.

After a few minutes, I notice lights outside the window. My first thought is that an ambulance is bringing in a patient, and the flashing lights are bouncing off the buildings across the street. Then I notice that the lights are green, blue, and yellow, not the red of ambulance lights. I am experiencing the aurora borealis, sometimes visible dancing in the sky over the prairies on cold nights.[7] He looks out the window, and we are watching the northern lights together.

He turns to look at me, tears streaming down his face, and says, "My ancestors have come to visit me." I realize that this is the time for me to leave his room so he can be alone with his dancing spirits in the sky.

The next day, the puzzle becomes clearer. His chart arrives from his previous hospitalization, where he was treated for his hip abscess. It was a *Staph aureus* infection, which required months of treatment and a long stay in the hospital. He has a background history of injection drug use, with the last use about two years ago, the chart says. Staph infection is difficult to eradicate and tends to harbour in the bone undetected for months, even after treatment is completed.

In the years since I met Michael, I have sometimes reflected on the moments that I sat at his bedside watching his ears fill with tears and the aurora borealis dancing before me. Soon after he was admitted to hospital, he underwent surgery on his leg and received a peripherally inserted central catheter (PICC) for ongoing intravenous antibiotics. When I visited him again in his private room on the orthopedic ward, we didn't talk about the tears, and we didn't dwell on why he was in jail. After five days he returned to the Regina Correctional Centre, receiving

---

7   The aurora borealis results from collisions of gaseous particles in the atmosphere. The solar wind takes charged particles from the sun and blows them towards the Earth. The Earth's magnetic field is weakest at the north pole; therefore, some particles from the sun enter the Earth's atmosphere. They collide with gas particles in the Earth's atmosphere and this produces lights—often green, blue, violet, yellow, or orange—in the sky.

ongoing treatment with antibiotics through their nursing station inside the jail. He had six weeks remaining on his sentence, the same amount of time that he will need the nursing station at the jail for his daily antibiotics.

I made a feeble attempt to visit him in jail and ran into a roadblock. If I were a family member, it would not be a problem, but I would require special permission even as a physician. I was told it would take months of paperwork. As I write this in 2023, I have never seen Michael again. I don't know if he got out of jail, or got killed in jail, if he is working in the mainstream, or living on his home reserve. I do know that if he is alive, he will always walk with a limp. I know that I will always remember him.

AN HIV EPIDEMIC

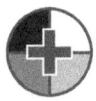

Bill, a fifty-six-year-old resident of the reserve, walks into the examination room of the health clinic wearing a neatly starched plaid shirt, blue jeans, cowboy boots, and a buckskin jacket with fringe. His salt-and-pepper hair is cut short in front, but he wears a long, neat braid down his back. I've known Bill for a couple of years; I tell him this morning that he looks like a fashionable version of the Indian scout, ready to ride out and explore the wide prairie.

Bill has hypertension, or high blood pressure, a disease that is common in both the settler and Indigenous populations. There are several possible causes—for example, atherosclerosis, kidney disease, or high hormones. Most of the time, no cause is found; doctors use the term *idiopathic*, which means we know that something is going on but not why. Hypertension can happen at any age, but it's more common with aging as the blood vessels harden. Untreated, it can damage the kidneys and cause strokes or heart disease.

Stress often increases blood pressure. In North America's academic and tech circles many people are enrolling in mindfulness meditation classes to treat hypertension without the use of drugs. Bill's blood pressure is up today, and he tells me he has been dealing with a lot of stress. I look him in the eyes and ask: "What's going on?"

His manner turns serious. "My daughter was living in Regina and got mixed up with some bad shit," he says. "She finally left the guy that she was living with, supposedly, and moved back home to reserve. She has two little kids who need taking care of. They're all living with me and my wife, but things are not smooth."

"Why not?" I ask. I'm trying to determine if stress is causing his blood pressure to rise, or if the medication that he's taking needs to change.

"I'm worried," he says. "When I was a teenager, I left reserve and moved into the city. I got mixed up with some bad players. I never went to jail, but I know the scene." I sit quietly on my stool close to the exam table facing him. Without him explicitly telling me, I understand that he's talking about drugs.

"Her boyfriend is part of a gang. There's a group of them coming on to the reserve. We can't leave the house and go shopping. There've been break-ins when people go to the city for shopping or to see a doctor. I've told my daughter to stop any contact with this guy, but I think she is still using. She leaves for days at a time. The kids stay with us. I sleep with a shotgun under my bed."

Bill appears calm and composed, but he is struggling with a terrifying reality. I feel my own heartbeat accelerating in response. I focus on breathing slowly as a way to maintain an emotional distance. There are so many people in distress here: the patient, his wife, a daughter whose life has spun out of control, two small children, and everyone on reserve who is affected by this outbreak of violence. I have no doubt that Bill is experiencing repeated eruptions of cortisol, the hormone associated with the body's flight-or-fight response. Our bodies react to increased cortisol levels in a variety of ways, and in this case it is affecting his blood pressure.

As I constantly remind myself during these consultations, I can't solve the issues that are creating my patient's stress. I can only treat the effects. I double his blood pressure medication on a temporary basis and ask him to monitor his blood pressure at home. I ask him to come back in a month.

"And before you go," I add, "there's something else." This is important; it could be life or death. If his daughter is sharing needles and engaging in high-risk sex, there is a high probability that she has contracted HIV or Hepatitis C, or both. Either infection is potentially fatal if left untreated. I tell him I'm available to see his daughter if she is willing to come, or I can arrange to have another doctor or a nurse see her, either here or in the city. But she needs testing *now*.

"Thanks, Dr. Boan," he says. "I'll let her know." Unfortunately, I will never meet Bill's daughter.

+ + +

In 2015, *Maclean's* magazine published an article about Saskatchewan's HIV epidemic that brought national attention to an issue that had troubled Saskatchewan's public health and infectious disease specialists for years.[1] The province had seen an increasing incidence of cases on reserve, among urban people who used IV drugs, and in hospitalized Indigenous patients. Physicians had recognized the HIV epidemic before the statistics appeared. They could see the patients sitting in front of them. We hadn't seen this volume of patients with HIV infection—a preventable and treatable condition—since the first wave of AIDS (acquired immune deficiency syndrome) in the 1980s.

The human immunodeficiency virus (HIV) is an infection that inhibits the body's immune system. It targets CD4 and T cell lymphocytes and allows unusual infections to invade the body. A 2015 article in the

---

[1] Ken MacQueen, "Saskatchewan's HIV Epidemic: Third World Levels of HIV Infection Rates in One of the World's Wealthiest Countries Are 'a National Disgrace,'" *Maclean's*, July 22, 2015, https://macleans.ca/news/canada/saskatchewans-hiv-epidemic/.

Canadian Medical Association Journal—an article that may have triggered the *Maclean's* report—stated that "according to Health Canada, the rate of new infections on reserves was 64 per 100,000 people at last count. That is nearly 11 times the national average of 5.9 per 100,000, and rivals nations like Nigeria and Rwanda."[2]

My colleague Dr. Alex Wong presented similar data at the 2015 International AIDS Society Conference on HIV Pathogenesis, Treatment and Prevention in Vancouver. His presentation, "The Developing World in Our Own Backyard: Concentrated HIV Epidemics in High Income Settings," referred to higher income nations such as Canada, the US, Australia, and the countries of Western Europe. Dr. Wong had studied case rates in communities surrounding Indigenous reserves. He reported that 80 percent of new HIV cases in Saskatchewan were occurring among Indigenous people. Making the same comparison as the author of the *CMAJ* piece, he used the phrase "Africa in the Prairies."

The funding situation in Saskatchewan improved only very slowly, based partly on the ease of accessibility of HIV medications. The odds for successful treatment jumped in 2006 with the development of a single tablet that could be taken once daily. As of 2021, we estimated that two-thirds of the HIV-positive patients identified in Saskatchewan had received treatment. Patients who look after themselves—who avoid using dirty needles, dodge other non-HIV infections, and show up for their medical appointments—now stand a good chance of living a normal life span. The problem now lies with the unidentified patients—the ones that do not go for HIV testing.

Another obstacle arose during the COVID pandemic, when access to HIV testing was reduced by the movement of public health staff from

---

2   Lauren Vogel, "HIV in Saskatchewan Merits Urgent Response," *Canadian Medical Association Journal* 187, no. 11 (Aug 11, 2015): 793–794, https://doi.org/10.1503/cmaj.109-5105.

community work to vaccine administration. Many patients confessed that they didn't want to access any health services during COVID and stayed away from clinics and hospitals. A report from local HIV network All Nations Hope's research director Margaret Kisikaw Piyesis raised concerns about the shutdown of public health clinics, addiction services, and shelters during the pandemic.[3] These closures and avoidances resulted in a jump in HIV cases that went untreated, the majority of them in the Indigenous population. Saskatchewan was front page news again in 2022 with the highest rate of HIV in Canada.[4]

Unfortunately, the Saskatchewan HIV epidemic is associated with a second complex infection associated with IV drug use and blood transfusions. Hepatitis C was first identified in 1989 as a virus linked to liver disease. Early studies indicated that perhaps 20 percent of people who were infected spontaneously recovered without treatment. For those who did not, the virus was often silent for many years, and because the symptoms were initially mild, Hepatitis C was difficult to diagnose. Detection depended on a targeted blood test; if neither the doctor nor the patient suspected Hepatitis C, they would be unlikely to ask for the test.

Around the late 1990s in Saskatchewan, the medical community began seeing people with liver fibrosis and started looking for evidence of Hepatitis C. They discovered it in a range of populations, including middle-aged people with a history of casual heroin use in their youth and hardcore current users of IV drugs. The extent of infection specifically in the Indigenous population was difficult to discern since

---

3   Mah Noor Mubarik, "HIV Cases Increased in Sask. with Pandemic Closures, Indigenous Organization Says," CBC News, December 6, 2021, https://www.cbc.ca/news/canada/saskatchewan/hiv-help-people-1.6275755.
4   Zosia Bielski, "STIs Spreading Aggressively in Canada as Testing, Prevention Abandoned During Pandemic," *The Globe and Mail*, April 8, 2022, https://www.theglobeandmail.com/canada/article-stis-rise-across-canada-after-limited-access-to-testing-and-treatment/.

provincial data collection does not ask about race or ethnicity. However, reports of frequent Hepatitis C infection among groups at high risk for HIV, such as provincial prison inmates and clients at needle exchange clinics, proliferated, and Indigenous people make up an oversized share of both these groups. As a result of these reports, the specific Hepatitis C blood test was added to the screening program for HIV; it turned out that Saskatchewan had another epidemic to deal with, again one that primarily affects Indigenous people.

Overall in Canada, it was estimated in 2019 that 338,000 people were infected with the Hepatitis C virus, most of them between thirty and fifty-five years of age.[5] The resulting disease is one of middle age that may appear many years after the person carrying the virus has abandoned their high-risk behaviour. Indigenous people in Canada were seven times more likely to be infected with Hepatitis C compared with those in the general population: it was estimated in 2019 that 13,400 (or 7.0 percent) of Indigenous people were infected with Hepatitis C, and 11 percent of incarcerated persons had Hepatitis C.[6] The infection was more prevalent in Saskatchewan than nationally.

Some academic papers on Hepatitis C focus on the financial cost of leaving the disease untreated and the need for preventive measures, which include early screening, providing harm-reduction programs in communities at risk, developing safe injection facilities, and providing treatment to active injection drug users to prevent onward Hep C transmission. The pharmaceutical industry has responded with improved treatments over time, but the price tag is high.

---

5 E. Payne, S. Totten, and C. Archibald, "Hepatitis C Surveillance in Canada," *Canada Communicable Disease Report* 40, no. 19 (December 18, 2014): 421–428, https://doi.org/10.14745/ccdr.v40i19a01.

6 Public Health Agency of Canada, "People Living with Hepatitis C (HCV) in Canada, 2019," Government of Canada, https://www.canada.ca/en/public-health/services/publications/diseases-conditions/infographic-people-living-with-hepatitis-c.html.

Communicable infections like HIV and Hepatitis C are preventable and strongly linked to the social determinants of health such as housing, education, and income levels. If you don't have a stable housing situation, you are less likely to get to the pharmacy for your HIV or Hep C drugs. If you are poor and you face a choice between food and medicine, you will choose food. As I have described in this book, some of my patients are people who have struggled with addiction and with the health effects of random, unsupervised drug use. I direct these patients to whatever treatment is available. However, to be honest, our medical treatments are often no more effective than applying a bandage. Until our communities can improve the underlying health determinants, I predict that we will continue to see high rates of infection leading to chronic disease and increased drug overdoses leading to death.

A CLINIC IN THE PARKLANDS

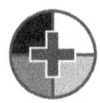

On an August morning in 2018, my phone dings with a text from Stu: *don't ring the doorbell, the dogs go crazy.* It is 6:00 a.m., the sun is up, the prairies show a sparkling tinge of morning dew. My taxi arrives at Stu's house on the east side of Regina fifteen minutes later. He's waiting in his SUV in the driveway. I have my stethoscope and overnight bag, and I climb in beside him. First stop is Tim Hortons for coffee.

It's a five-hour drive to our destination, north and west from the Wascana Plains to the edge of the deep forest. We will pick up our colleague JoLee in Saskatoon and travel the final three hours to the territory of the Ahtahkakoop Cree Nation. This is where Stu first began practising medicine on reserve, honing his focus on HIV and Hepatitis C, in the days before Wellness Wheel. As resident of Saskatoon, he developed a long-term relationship with this reserve. His experience helped him design the concept of Wellness Wheel. We will participate in an afternoon clinic, drive for an hour to the city of Prince Albert to stay overnight in a hotel, and then return to Ahtahkakoop for another half day.

As we drive, our conversation turns to big ideas for change. Stu asks me to lay out my solutions for Indigenous health. We know the problems: poverty, lack of access to care, institutions that fail to consult with each other, transfer payments with strings attached, lack of band resources to build water systems and child care, lack of housing.

In the end, I have to say that I am not hopeful that we will find solutions. Improvement, perhaps, and possibly the elimination of some mindless obstacles and a reduction in the frequency of lethal effects. To agree on any course of action, we need to keep reviewing, revisiting, and rehashing our understanding of what ails the health care system.

On the drive to Ahtahkakoop from Saskatoon, we have time to talk with JoLee, someone I have never spoken with on a personal level before. She is a bright and engaging forty-year-old woman. She tells us her life story from the back seat of the car. Her husband is a member of the Ahtahkakoop Cree Nation. She is Ojibwa from Ontario and grew up in Northern Michigan. Through a circuitous route, she completed a PhD and became a researcher at a university. She is a key speaker for OCAP (the organization devoted to the protection of Indigenous data).

She expresses her frustration with housing on reserve. The Chief decides on the housing priorities. There is a waiting list at Ahtahkakoop; JoLee's husband's application for housing has not yet been approved. The couple lives in a cabin on his father's property on reserve, without running water. Understandably, she is vocal in expressing her opinions about local politics.

The flat prairie changes to rolling bush. This was the land of the beaver and a reliable trading area for the Hudson's Bay Company before the settlers arrived. The Métis had a strong presence along the North Saskatchewan River until they were excluded from treaty signing, displaced from their land, and forced to squat on road allowances. With a marginalized existence and the decline of the beaver fur trade, the

Métis people's lives were as dismal as those of their fellow hunters who were placed on reserves.

We arrive at the Ahtahkakoop Health Centre just after noon. It is a modern building with a waiting room, multiple offices, exam rooms, computers, counselling rooms, a kitchen, and a large meeting space. Outside, there's a marked landing pad for helicopters, allowing clinic staff to airlift patients to Saskatoon or Regina. We enter through the back door into a kitchen that doubles as a meeting room, where we find twenty people seated around a large oval table. Noreen Reed, the Health Director and our host, greets us with a smile. The group has been enjoying a home-cooked meal, and they invite us to eat with them. After introductions, we load up paper plates with fried chicken, mashed potatoes, and fresh green beans, and engage in a conversation about the health centre's patient load and patient flow.

Throughout the afternoon, I become familiar with the diabetes cases. Stu looks at the Hepatitis C and HIV case load, and JoLee visits with her husband's family and other members of the Nation.

This Ahtahkakoop facility, to our minds, presents fewer organizational problems than we see farther south. The patients arrive for their appointments on time through a system organized by Noreen, who has a driver pick them up at their homes and deliver them to the clinic. A big part of the health centre's focus is on diabetic patients; funding for nurses, diabetes educators, and a pharmacist is paid for from federal Indigenous Services Canada funding for diabetes care. But for me, the most memorable interaction from that day is unrelated to diabetes.

The patient is an active member of the community, whom I'll call Wayne. He sits before me in a blue button-down shirt and nicely pressed jeans. He wears a carved leather belt at his waist, with a shiny engraved buckle, and cowboy boots. His straight dark hair is cut short. He has no facial hair. His dark eyes look into my hazel eyes, and he begins to cry.

The relationship between a doctor and patient is sacred. People confess things to a doctor that they don't tell other people. This trust is a first step in the healing process, and a powerful force for people in need of help. I can't tell you any more about Wayne. His identity and reputation may depend on the dark secret that he reveals to me: he is addicted to heroin.

As usual, I don't ask too many questions, but let him talk between sobs. Over the previous year, he has hooked up with a woman from another reserve, and she recently moved in with him. As the relationship developed and became more intimate, so did the need for some excitement. It started slowly with the occasional use of heroin to get high together and to laugh with drug-induced euphoria. We sometimes call this *dabbling*. These experiments enhanced Wayne's confidence and increased his ability to converse with others. His alertness increased, and he ventured into a different dimension of intimacy with his friends and family. He enjoyed it, and so did his girlfriend, who initiated the slide from social use into dependency with more frequent use. "I just found myself wanting more and more. I'd put the pipe down, and then two hours later I'd want it again. I'd wake up in the morning and want more," Wayne says, his head hung low. His job on reserve suffered. His girlfriend left him and moved out. He was depressed and recognized that he needed help.

After telling me his story, Wayne stops crying and looks up at me. He has a goal in mind, and he believes that I can help him.

Nearby the Ahtahkakoop Health Centre is the Cree Nations Treatment Haven, the first of its kind in Saskatchewan. Housed in a separate building of log construction, it allows people struggling with addictions to participate in a culturally appropriate treatment program. Services include multidisciplinary addictions management, a five-week residential detox course, and a sixteen-week outpatient treatment course. Twice each month, a team made up of a physician, nurse, and counsellor visits from the Prince Albert medical community. The team approach helps to determine the type of treatment that new patients require, including the question of whether treatment should take place in hospital or in the community. In between the health team visits, the program is managed by local recovered patients who distribute methadone or Suboxone on a daily basis to those struggling with addiction on reserve.

A harm reduction program using opioid agonist therapy is not the antidote for addiction, but it provides users with a respite from craving while they focus on changing their addictive habits and understanding the root causes of their addiction.[1] The health centre conducts weekly urine screens on each patient who is registered for the on-reserve program. Many patients struggle even when they have access to opioid substitutes, and they use illicit drugs intermittently. The urine tests often show multiple substances, including gabapentin, benzos (benzodiazepine tranquilizers), THC (marijuana), morphine, hydromorphone, alcohol, cocaine, and crystal meth. The goal of treatment is to keep patients off the daily use of street drugs and have them experience reality without the use of mind-altering drugs. When a urine test comes back positive for illicit drugs, the counsellor and the physician meet with the patient and remind them of the rules: a couple of slip-ups are permissible, but continued drug use will disqualify them, and they will be barred from the harm reduction program program.

A pharmacy in Prince Albert provides the opioid agonists (methadone or Suboxone) through physicians' prescriptions. The medication travels to reserve in secure metal boxes, and the volume of each

---

[1] "POLICY—Opioid Agonist Therapy (OATP) Prescribing," College of Physicians and Surgeons of Saskatchewan, November 2018, https://www.cps.sk.ca/imis/CPSS/CPSS/Legislation__ByLaws__Policies_and_Guidelines/Legislation_Content/Policies_and_Guidelines_Content/OAT_Prescribing.aspx.

shipment is accounted for as it is deposited in the treatment centre, where it is kept under lock and key. Monitoring of the treatment centre and its contents is provided by former participants in the program, following the accepted principle that the best role-modelling in treatment programs is peer-based.[2] A community member who is no longer using drugs shares a community with the person who is struggling. They share a common culture, language, and experience. Peer-based medical programs sometimes use other names to describe the role of a peer: community health workers, health coaches, lay health advisors, patient navigators, or doulas.[3] In the medical literature, other examples of peer-based approaches include using peers to address treatment of asthma, diabetes, cancer, HIV/AIDS, smoking cessation, breast self-exam, condom use, and mental health support. This approach has been shown to be cost effective and especially successful in populations that are hard to reach or rural.[4] The Cree Nations Treatment Haven, using an Indigenous approach with collective shared knowledge, ceremonies, experiential relationships with nature, and spiritual reflection, to make it culturally adapted. They use miskâsowin, a Cree word that means to go to the centre of yourself to find your own belonging.[5]

---

[2] Allison R. Webel, Jennifer Okonsky, Joyce Trompeta, and William L. Holzemer, "A Systematic Review of the Effectiveness of Peer-Based Interventions on Health-Related Behaviors in Adults," *American Journal of Public Health* 100, no.2 (February 2010), 247–253, https://doi.org/10.2105/AJPH.2008.149419. See also: Canadian AIDS Society and the Canadian Harm Reduction Network, *Learning from Each Other: Enhancing Community-Based Harm Reduction Programs and Practices in Canada* (2008), https://www.cdnaids.ca/wp-content/uploads/Learning-from-Each-Other.pdf.

[3] Henry B. Perry, Rose Zulliger, and Michael M. Rogers, "Community Health Workers in Low-, Middle-, and High-Income Countries: An Overview of Their History, Recent Evolution, and Current Effectiveness," *Annual Review of Public Health* 35 (March 2014): 399–421, https://doi.org/10.1146/annurev-publhealth-032013-182354.

[4] Perry, Zulliger, and Rogers, "Community Health Workers: An Overview."

[5] Harold Cardinal and Walter Hildebrandt, "Miskâsowin Finding One's Sense of...

Once a patient stabilizes on a prescribed opioid agonists, they enter a maintenance routine for either long-term methadone use or self-weaning. Clinic staff report an increase in self-esteem with this reserve-based community program. Opioid agonists provide control. The caseload for this program was sixty Ahtahkakoop members as of 2020, and there was a waiting list for treatment.

Wayne has chosen me, as a visiting doctor, to get him into a treatment program without revealing his identity. If he wants to enter the Ahtahkakoop program, he must trust me enough to sign a form allowing me to speak with the treatment team. The alternative is a two-hour round trip to Prince Albert whenever he needs treatment, which might be every day.

The on-reserve program is effective and close by, but Wayne is afraid that if he is seen at the treatment centre, it will ruin his standing in the community. He chooses the Prince Albert option. I pick up the phone to make a contact, then write a referral that I will fax later from Regina. With a nurse, I prepare the glass tubes needed for standard HIV and Hep C screening, something the Prince Albert clinic will need before starting treatment. We have a plan in place. Wayne looks relieved as he leaves the exam room.

In follow-up, I learned that Wayne was negative for both HIV and Hepatitis C, so his addictions treatment would not be complicated by pills for these infections and their side effects. He was put on a daily regimen of methadone to control his cravings. After six months, he switched to Suboxone, ingesting one pill daily at home. Eventually this dose was tapered, and he broke free. Wayne has become a strong

---

…Origin and Belonging, Finding 'One's Self' or Finding 'One's Centre,'" in *Treaty Elders of Saskatchewan: Our Dream Is That Our Peoples Will One Day Be Clearly Recognized as Nations* (Calgary: University of Calgary Press, 2000), 21–24, https://doi.org/10.2307/j.ctv6gqwq3.11.

advocate for land-based, peer-led treatment among Saskatchewan Indigenous populations. His healing began with his ability to recognize his need for help, his willingness to confide in me, and his trust that I would not judge his tears.

At the end of our afternoon at the clinic, we join JoLee at her father-in-law's house on the edge of Sandy Lake. Fred Sasakamoose is former Chief of the Ahtahkakoop Nation and a retired hockey player and coach. The log house he shares with his wife is cool and inviting in the summer heat. His wife is Métis; she grew up in a cabin on a road allowance nearby. We look at photos on his living room walls showing him in a Chicago Black Hawks uniform holding the Stanley Cup, and at a lifetime's worth of awards and certificates related to his work on behalf of Indigenous youth and Indigenous participation in sport, and at his Order of Canada citation.

Fred talks about his time in residential school, remembering first that they cut his hair. He talks about the pain of coping with the strict rules and being separated from his family and culture. Then, he says, he was recruited for hockey, travelled all over Canada and the United States, and made friends of all kinds. He is proud but humble. I ask him whether his residential school experience acted as a barrier to his early success as a hockey player; he says, on the contrary, that his school years prepared him for immersion in the white world, and that he would never have succeeded in pro sports without his residential school education. Yet, the trauma of separation from his family and the loss of Indigenous culture is still painful for him.

He goes to a desk in the corner of the living room and returns to give us each a picture of himself in his Black Hawks jersey, on skates, holding a hockey stick, smiling. It is a gesture of hospitality we did not expect.

We thank him and then visit JoLee and Derrick's cabin, built a hundred yards from Fred's house, with a balcony that looks over the lake. The aspen and spruce forests of the north are golden, timeless, on a warm summer afternoon. After this restorative pause, we return to our hotel rooms through the evening light.

In November 2020, Fred Sasakamoose died of complications related to COVID-19. He was eighty-six years old.

"Fred Sasakamoose survived the residential school system, became the National Hockey League's first-ever Indigenous player and inspired many with his stories of suffering and success," Prime Minister Justin Trudeau said in a tribute on Twitter. "He leaves behind an incredible legacy."[6]

Before Fred passed away, just a few months after our visit, our hosts JoLee and Derrick Sasakamoose would teach me more lessons about the medicine chest clause and the legacy of Ahtahkakoop.

---

6   @JustinTrudeau, November 24, 2020, 8:29 p.m., https://twitter.com/JustinTrudeau/status/1331409684264349698.

DERRICK

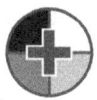

In my memory of a summer day in Northern Saskatchewan, Derrick Sasakamoose is a large, gentle man with the same grave politeness that I experienced with his father, Fred. However, there is an edge to Derrick, and I intuitively feel I would not want to provoke him. We shake hands outside his log cabin on the shores of Sandy Lake as the late afternoon sun warms us. His thumb is raised to the sun acknowledging the Creator as he extends his hand. His palm slaps into mine, and his fingers grasp my hand firmly. "We need our kinships to survive. We are all treaty people," he says, and I am welcomed to his ancestral homeland. I'm grateful. His smile is warm and welcoming as he shows Stu and me around his cabin.

We are introduced to him by his wife, JoLee, as the specialist doctors who have come to Ahtahkakoop to assist at the health clinic. I engage him in conversation unrelated to health. The log cabin, which has no running water or electricity, was given to them by Fred and is a summer home on his family's land. They intend to build a house on top of the hill. "Where do you get your drinking water?" I inquire, sounding like an urbanite with no wilderness survival abilities. "Is it cold in the evenings? How do you keep your food safe from the bears in the woods?"

He then tells me about the city doctors he has seen and how "they just do not listen to him." Carefully I say, "I'm here for another half day; you can come in and talk." He agrees to come to the on-reserve clinic the following day.

The following morning, when the health centre's doors open, I meet with people with diabetes who are dealing with several challenges, the most prevalent of which is being out of insulin. I am curious about the challenges patients are experiencing in keeping their insulin prescriptions filled, and the effectiveness of diabetes education, as this health clinic has a high level of community engagement. I am struck by the irony that insulin was discovered in Canada, yet it is not universally available to those who need it.

Derrick arrives at noon. In the exam room, he tells me that he's a recovering methadone addict, clean for several years. I ask if he would agree to have lab tests done to check his HIV and Hepatitis C status; he declines, suggesting that he does not like needles. I respect his boundaries and do not push him. Later, when I learn more about Derrick's experience, I wish I had been more assertive.

While I am visiting patients with diabetes and meeting with Derrick, Stu, the infectious disease specialist, is in another room performing HIV and Hepatitis C testing and treatment. Testing for these conditions necessitates the collection of a blood sample and an in-depth discussion with the patient to explain why a sample is required. It is crucial to check the patient's viral load and natural antibodies: up to 25 percent of patients will clear the Hepatitis C virus independently, while the rest will most likely need treatment. The testing methodology also requires us to assess the severity of liver damage, which we conduct using ultrasound equipment that assesses fibrosis. We bring the portable FibroScan machine to each "liver clinic." The scan is painless and offers quick results. In partnership with the community, we have collected data over time to understand the disease's impacts.

Untreated Hepatitis C–related liver disease frequently progresses to cirrhosis, liver failure, multiple hospitalizations, and possibly liver cancer. If a patient is fortunate, they will be referred for liver transplantation and placed on a lengthy waiting list. In 2014, the average lifetime cost of untreated Hepatitis C was estimated to be $64,694 without a liver transplant. Taxpayers bear these expenditures through provincial medical insurance programs. By comparison, the cost of a liver transplant in Canada was $237,608. It made sense to fund treatment and prevention of Hepatitis C rather than pay for liver transplants.[1]

Prior to 2000, the only drug we had for treating Hep C was interferon. It was given by injection, and the side effects were brutal. Patients receiving interferon needed careful monitoring with frequent lab tests, which was difficult on reserve where there was no easy access to a medical laboratory. On top of that, the cure rate was only 40 percent.

With the advent of an oral pill with fewer side effects and a better cure rate, life for everyone became easier. The problem was the cost. Wealthy Hollywood stars could afford to pay $84,000 out-of-pocket for the three-month course of treatment, but this price was prohibitive for the average person. Public health advocates initiated legal challenges to the pharmaceutical industry's patent claims, on the basis that this was a public health issue and lives were at risk. Governments that funded drug plans and formularies got involved to negotiate the price. Then, in 2014, there was an interesting twist about patent claims. The company that manufactured the drug sought approval for generic manufacturing

---

1   Robert P. Myers, Mel Krajden, Marc Bilodeau, Kelly Kaita, Paul Marotta, Kevork Peltekian, Alnoor Ramji, Chris Estes, Homie Razavi, and Morris Sherman, "Burden of Disease and Cost of Chronic Hepatitis C Infection in Canada," *Canadian Journal of Gastroenterology and Hepatology* 28 (2014): 243–250, https://doi.org/10.1155/2014/317623.

of the drug in overseas labs,[2] on the basis that the drug should be available in developing countries. They priced the three-month treatment cost at $8,939 in China in 2015.[3] This was the perfect opportunity for Indigenous Services Canada, the federal government department that manages the health of Indigenous populations, to advocate for treatment across Canada. By 2015, the drug's retail price—$20,000 for its three-month supply—was made affordable under the ISC's Non-Insured Health Benefits program at no cost to First Nation's patients. This was my first realization of the power of a national mandate for health treatment that superseded the provincial Medicare policies to make care available to all those who qualified. Unfortunately, since settler populations are covered by provincial Medicare programs, they were left out of the ISC mandate.

The year we visited Ahtahkakoop, federal government funders had just approved Hepatitis C treatment for Indigenous patients. They had recognized, finally, that the expense of allowing the disease to progress was greater than the twelve-week treatment cost. I could have initiated Derrick's treatment on that August day in Ahtahkakoop, but he declined to get tested, and I was unaware of his past experience.

JoLee called me on my Regina cellphone four months later and said Derrick had been "behaving strangely." His mind was cloudy, and he had trouble recalling previous conversations. He was perpetually sleeping. He felt ill and could not eat. Derrick and JoLee had moved with

---

2   Press release, "Gilead Announces Generic Licensing Agreements to Increase Access to to Hepatitis C Treatments in Developing Countries," Gilead, September 15, 2014, https://www.gilead.com/news-and-press/press-room/press-releases/2014/9/gilead-announces-generic-licensing-agreements-to-increase-access-to-hepatitis-c-treatments-in-developing-countries.

3   Arlene Weintraub, "Gilead Prices Hepatitis C Giant Sovaldi in China at One-Fifth the US Price: Report," Fierce Pharma, November 28, 2017, https://www.fiercepharma.com/financials/gilead-prices-hep-c-giant-sovaldi-china-at-one-fifth-u-s-price-report.

their son to spend the academic year in Regina, where JoLee was working as a professor. I invited her to bring Derrick to my Albert Street office, and they arrived within thirty minutes. I was surprised to see a pale and ashen man, his complexion tinged with yellow.

I asked him a few questions even before he sat down: "Do you have black stools? Are you spitting up blood? Are you having trouble peeing? Do you suffer from chest pain?" If he had answered yes to these questions, I would have rushed him to the Emergency Room. He said no, but his responses were sluggish and monosyllabic. His blood pressure was high, and he had swelling in his face, arms, and legs. I suspected fluid in his abdomen, but he did not seem to be in any pain when I touched him. I persisted in my proposal that we run lab tests, and this time Derrick agreed. I phoned the Regina General ER and informed them that Derrick would require lab work and X-rays.

We paused for a moment to allow the paperwork to clear the hospital's system, and I posed one last question: "Have you ever been tested for Hepatitis C?"

"Yes," he said, and he had tested positive.

"When did you discover this?" I pressed.

"Two years ago in Regina, but I cured it with traditional medicine on reserve," he replied, looking me in the eyes.

JoLee, sitting in the corner of my office, slumped in her chair. Derrick had never told her he was positive for Hep C. She sat for several minutes with tears streaming down her face.

That evening, an ER doctor called me from the hospital with bad news. Derrick's kidney function was disturbed and his liver enzymes were sky high. He was in liver failure. His test for Hep C was positive.

I drove to the hospital from my home. I found JoLee sitting in the hallway outside Derrick's room, still crying. I invited her into a small conference room nearby. We sat across from each other at the table, and I asked her to tell me what she knew.

Several years before this, while she was working in Sioux Lookout in Northern Ontario and living with her adoptive family, they invited her to attend a Sweat Ceremony on the Ahtahkakoop Cree Nation in Saskatchewan. The night before they began the long drive, she had vivid dreams and sensed something spiritual was coming. When she and her adoptive father arrived at the Ahtahkakoop Sweat Lodge, Derrick was the first person she met. He had been serving as an oskâpêwis (Sweat Lodge or Elder's helper). There was instant chemistry. They chatted and exchanged numbers.

Derrick and JoLee communicated for several months before William, her adoptive father, returned with her to Ahtahkakoop. William was a friend of Derrick's father, Fred, and they talked in Cree for hours in front of Fred's wood stove. Then they called JoLee and Derrick and told the two younger people that they were being matched. The Elders spoke with them at length about the life issues they might face. JoLee was thirty-nine and Derrick was forty-six; they both respected the traditional ways and were willing to give the relationship a chance. Derrick admitted to a past of drug misuse, but he was now clean. He agreed to drive JoLee back to Sioux Lookout.

Two years later, they married on Lonesome Pine Hill in Ahtahkakoop. JoLee got a job as a professor in Regina, and they bought a house. She became pregnant and had a healthy baby boy. Derrick worked for the Truth and Reconciliation Commission in their Resolution Health Support Program. He spent his days in hearings, serving as cultural support to residential school Survivors who recounted their experiences of rape, torture, witnessing murder, and abuse while attending residential schools. After two years of listening to traumatic testimony, Derrick's behaviour began to change. JoLee could see the change and questioned him about it. He admitted to relapsing. He progressively declined, and then he left their home.

Derrick was missing for several months while JoLee struggled as a single working mom. When she decided to sell their house and move to something smaller, she realized she would need his signature. She called his family. He's in Regina, they said, but he had only contacted them to ask for money.

She drove around in search of Derrick and noticed his car sitting in front of a house in North Central. She knocked, and Derrick's cousin answered and let her in. It was a drug house, and she discovered Derrick lying on a mattress on the floor, rumpled and filthy. He raised his eyes to her, embarrassed. She felt empathy for the father of her son. She said that their child needed his father, and she offered to take him to detox. He refused. Months went by. Periodically, JoLee would locate Derrick and offer the same lifeline: a ride to treatment, a visit with their son, a ray of hope.

Derrick was bitten by a spider one day and came perilously near death while receiving treatment in hospital. After surviving this experience, he went to detox, feeling the Creator had given him a second opportunity. He then moved on to a course of treatment at Pine Lodge just south of the Qu'Appelle Valley. He would never use drugs again, but his body was harbouring a silent killer. The health care system would fail him.

With JoLee's consent and participation, he began to visit with their son in a local park. He stayed sober, and she invited him to move into the basement of their house to act as a father to their son. He was a capable parent, assisting JoLee in her role as a working mother. Their marriage had changed, but they remained best friends and devoted parents, raising their son in the traditional way. They took a semester off to live on their land in Ahtahkakoop, and JoLee was confident that everything would be okay. Tragically, that was not to be.

When I met Derrick on my visit to the Parklands in Saskatchewan, he did not disclose that he was enrolled in a methadone program. Derrick and JoLee presented as a close, loving couple.

After my discussion with JoLee in the hospital conference room, I went to Derrick's bedside and asked him what had happened to him after he left Pine Lodge's treatment program. JoLee had told me he had seen a family doctor in Regina who gave him regular prescriptions of methadone. If there was a positive Hep C test result in Derrick's record, this doctor should have been aware of it.

I started slowly with Derrick. "I know Dr. X is your doctor," I said. "Did he ever ask about your Hepatitis C status?"

"Dr. X just gave me my methadone," he replied. "Every day, I had to go to his drugstore. He threatened me and warned me not to see another doctor. I went for a blood test and took the result to a public health nurse. She told me I had Hepatitis. I decided to use traditional medicines. When I told Dr. X, he got angry and told me it was a stupid decision. But he told me to go ahead. He didn't care."

In other words, this doctor threw up his hands and did not provide a constructive reply when confronted with an Indigenous patient who passed on the opportunity to get a proven medical cure. Instead, he simply lost his temper. In an earlier chapter, I mentioned how common it is for doctors to have poor communication skills. In Derrick's case, poor communication led to an outcome that was disastrous in a way I have seen only a few times in my thirty years of practice. The patient viewed the situation with mistrust, but his skepticism was well founded.

If Dr. X had started Derrick on treatment for Hepatitis C earlier, Derrick's liver might have been saved. By the time Derrick landed in the hospital in Regina, it was too late. I asked him, "If you knew that you were Hepatitis C positive, why didn't you tell JoLee?"

He lowered his eyes, "I was ashamed," he said, and began to cry. I felt my insides twist in empathy and anger.

Forty-eight hours after our meeting in my office, the hospital confirmed that Derrick's Hepatitis had caused his liver failure. He was flown to Edmonton and evaluated as a possible candidate for an emergency transplant. Soon after his arrival, he went into a coma. His family, including JoLee, drove to Edmonton and stayed in a hotel near the hospital. After four days, the doctors reported that his liver failure had caused too much damage to his other organs for him to survive surgery. They told JoLee that Derrick would be flown back so he could get stronger before being reevaluated for transplant, but it is likely the transfer was intended to bring him closer to home at the end of his life. Still in a coma, on a ventilator, Derrick was transported back to the Regina General ICU, where he died a few hours later.

At about this time, I learned the College of Physicians and Surgeons, the licensing authority for Saskatchewan doctors, was reviewing the records of harm reduction physicians. Nursing my anger about Derrick's death, I wrote to the college describing my experience with the patient and my suspicions about how his condition had been ignored. Policies state that to prescribe methadone, a physician is "required to try to provide non-pharmacological support to their patients (e.g., addiction services, counselling, harm reduction, community programs, etc.), and monitor laboratory results."[4]

A few months later, Dr. X lost his licence to prescribe methadone.

Harm reduction physicians must support their patients in moving away from opioid addiction. The problem, however, is that physicians can charge a fee for prescribing either methadone or Suboxone. Further, they can collect payment for every visit the methadone user takes to the pharmacy if they observe that the patient has taken their medication. Putting the pharmacy billings with back-to-back five-minute consults, a doctor who runs this kind of revolving door can make over $3,000 per day.

The College of Physicians and Surgeons review was intended to clamp down on lucrative methadone clinics to improve the quality of care. They gathered detailed intelligence on each doctor that they targeted.

---

4   "POLICY—Opioid Agonist Therapy (OATP) Prescribing," College of Physicians and Surgeons of Saskatchewan.

I will never know if my letter influenced their decision.

I felt no sense of triumph about reporting a doctor who appeared to use his practice to maximize profit at the expense of his patients. I was angry at first, then subsequently felt sadness and guilt for what happened to Derrick. We are hampered by a system that collects patient information sporadically, where clinicians may find it challenging to understand the big picture or may never make an effort. I feel frustration with a system where clinicians and Indigenous patients may be strangers, separated by a chasm of past trauma and mistrust.

This chapter was co-authored with Dr. JoLee Sasakamoose.

THE TRADE IN ALCOHOL

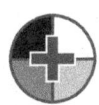

My medical practice in Regina consists of the treatment of patients in hospital and subsequent continued care in an outpatient setting. On a summer evening, I've made the easy ten-minute commute from my house on the south side of the city to the Regina General Hospital. Paramedics wheel an Indigenous patient into the ER; the police have found her collapsed on a downtown sidewalk. She is unconscious, unable to speak, but breathing. The intake nurse turns to me and says, "Another drunk one." I flinch at the racially induced snub.

This is how I met Sylvia, a forty-six-year-old Indigenous woman from a small reserve on the southern prairies. Her community is known among medical professionals for dysfunction, addiction, and troubled family circumstances. Not coincidentally, they had been uprooted from their traditional territory at the time of the nineteenth-century treaties and transported hundreds of miles to a desolate, treeless section of land that was of no value to the settlers.

Sylvia has been living in a spare room in a friend's house in North Central. At this moment, as she lies on a hospital gurney in a hallway, she is unconscious with a blood alcohol level of 282 mg/dl[1] and bleeding from her nose. Sylvia would later confide in me as I got to know her over the next five years, and I would grow to want to be the doctor who helped Sylvia save herself.

We keep Sylvia on her gurney until her alcohol level subsides, and then we let her go. Two weeks later she arrives at the ER complaining of intermittent nosebleeds. She requires packing, blood transfusion, and hospitalization. She has lost a lot of blood and become anemic. Her tendency to bleed has been worsened by her lack of blood clotting factors. Her INR (a measure of her liver function and ability to produce factors that help blood clotting) is elevated, at 1.6. Our test shows, in fact, that her liver is failing. We give her vitamin K to reverse her tendency to bleed, but an abdominal ultrasound of the liver shows a nodular surface, consistent with cirrhosis. Her spleen is enlarged. Since there are causes other than alcohol for liver cirrhosis, we test her for those diseases and she proves to be negative for both Hepatitis C and HIV. Under our treatment, and without the alcohol that was poisoning her liver, her bleeding stops.

Cirrhosis is the final pathway for most forms of liver disease. It is defined as a loss of functioning liver cells, which have been replaced by fibrous scarring. As the liver cells lose function, metabolic function is lost and toxins accumulate in the bloodstream. This produces a confused mental state that we call hepatic encephalopathy. The scarring reduces blood flow through the liver and creates backup pressure in all the vessels that flow into the liver. This results in internal bleeding from engorged vessels. Through a complicated loss of hormonal signaling in the liver, fluid accumulates in the abdominal cavity. We call this ascites.

---

[1] Blood alcohol level measurements are frequently used in the ER. A blood alcohol level of 80 mg/dl is equivalent to 0.08 on a breathalyzer test.

Sylvia is admitted to the hospital, and I check on her the next day. She confesses that she is an alcoholic and had been binge drinking. She agrees to speak with someone in the Native Health Services office at the hospital, and based on that meeting, she is booked to go to the Pine Lodge Treatment Centre in Indian Head, east of Regina, for two weeks of detox and rehabilitation.

We arrange an appointment for her to visit me in my office after she returns from the treatment centre. She does not show up. I hoped that the alcohol rehab program worked, that she was free from alcohol and didn't need my medical help. I wouldn't see her for a year.

Alcohol, notoriously, is a prominent actor in the story of how Canadian settlement has affected Indigenous people. Rum and whisky came to North America with the fur trade. The North West Company, the first major fur trading company to be based in Canada, raised the marketing of alcohol to a high art.² Canoes laden with barrels of alcohol were distributed from Fort William (now amalgamated into the city of Thunder Bay) on the western shore of Lake Superior throughout the Great Northwest—what is now Manitoba, Saskatchewan, and Alberta as well as the Dakotas and Montana. By some estimates, liquor consumption at the height of the fur trade was estimated to be fifty thousand gallons of distilled product per year.³ Diluted with water, the total reached 250,000 gallons for trading. Canoes would return along the riverways back to Fort William every spring laden with beaver furs. In

---

2   Marjorie Wilkins Campbell, *The North West Company* (Toronto: MacMillan Company, 1957). The North West Company figures prominently in the history of Canadian exploration (Alexander Mackenzie, David Thompson, Simon Fraser) as well as the exploitation of Indigenous people.
3   Harold R. Johnson, *Firewater: How Alcohol Is Killing My People (And Yours)* (Regina: University of Regina Press, 2016), 15.

some ways, this pattern resembled the structure of the modern illicit drug trade.[4]

In Canada in 2011, close to 80 percent of the general population over the age of fifteen consumed alcohol at least occasionally.[5] Federal statistics suggest that a slightly lower proportion of people living on reserve consumed alcohol, but three-quarters of people on reserve considered alcohol to be a problem in their communities.[6] Easy access to alcohol has made alcohol-related disease a leading cause of hospitalization in Canada for all demographic groups. In 2015–16, there were more hospitalizations due to alcohol than for heart attacks.[7] The Canadian Centre on Substance Use and Addiction (CCSA) reported that in 2014 more than 14,000 deaths in Canada were attributable to alcohol,[8] from motor vehicle accidents, homicides, domestic violence, suicide, liver failure, and alcohol-related cancer. Columnist and famous Canadian public health physician Trevor Hancock wrote in 2017 that if we want to save lives, we should exert more control over the sale and consumption of alcohol.[9]

---

4   Andrew Cockburn and Leslie Cockburn, writers and directors, *Frontline*, 613, "Guns, Drugs, and the CIA," original air date: May 17, 1988, PBS.
5   Gregory Taylor, "The Chief Public Health Officer's Report on the State of Public Health in Canada, 2015: Alcohol Consumption in Canada," www.canada.ca/en/public-health/services/publications/chief-public-health-officer-reports-state-public-health-canada/2015-alcohol-consumption-canada.html.
6   Saman Khan, "Aboriginal Mental Health: The Statistical Reality," *Visions Journal* 5, no. 1, Aboriginal People issue (Summer 2008): 6–7.
7   *Alcohol Harm in Canada* was released by the Canadian Institute for Health Information (CIHI). In Canada, alcohol is the top risk factor for disease among Canadians aged fifteen to forty-nine, according to the 2015 report from the chief public health officer.
8   Canadian Centre on Substance Use and Addiction, "Alcohol: Canadian Drug Summary," Report, Summer 2019, https://www.ccsa.ca/sites/default/files/2020-10/CCSA-Canadian-Drug-Summary-Alcohol-2019-en.pdf.
9   Trevor Hancock, "Trevor Hancock: If We Want to Save Lives, Control Alcohol," *Times Colonist*, July 15, 2017, https://www.timescolonist.com/opinion/trevor-...

The CCSA reported that the direct health care costs of alcohol in 2014 amounted to about $4.2 billion, and the total cost to the economy was more than $14.6 billion, almost half due to lost productivity. These numbers are conservative; in 2016, the chief public health officer's report on the state of public health in Canada reported that the full health and social costs of impaired driving alone in 2010 (including alcohol and other drugs) amounted to more than $20 billion.[10] Tax revenue from alcohol sales contributed approximately $12.8 billion to government revenues in Canada in 2020.[11]

Studies of alcoholism, or alcohol use disorder, show the risk factors to be exposure to aggressive behaviour in childhood, lack of parental supervision, poor social skills, poverty, and the availability of alcohol. Women and those with anxiety or depression are at higher risk for alcohol dependency. A recent report makes it clear that the prevalence of alcohol-related harm in society is directly related to price and availability. Paradoxically, those with limited incomes are twice as likely to be hospitalized with alcohol-related diseases, when compared to higher income patients hospitalized with alcohol-related conditions.[12] This paradox of hospitalization from alcohol use is thought to be related to better social support and diets, and lower levels of stress in the high-income patients. Increasing the price of alcohol will not necessarily eliminate the spread of alcohol-related diseases, but it will reduce consumption especially in heavy drinkers.

...hancock-if-we-want-to-save-lives-control-alcohol-4651433.

10   Taylor, "The Chief Public Health Officer's Report on the State of Public Health in Canada, 2015."
11   "Control and Sale of Alcoholic Beverages, Year Ending March 31, 2020," Statistics Canada, April 21, 2021, https://www150.statcan.gc.ca/n1/daily-quotidien/210421/dq210421b-eng.htm.
12   "The Alcohol Harm Paradox," Canadian Institiute for Health Information, 2918, https://www.cihi.ca/en/infographic-the-alcohol-harm-paradox.

Medical schools teach their students to recognize what is called alcohol use disorder. The diagnostic process is called the CAGE criteria, adapted to include drug use. Every medical student learns to ask questions about patterns of use, such as: Have you ever had a drink or used drugs first thing in the morning to steady your nerves or to get rid of a hangover?

The CAGE questionnaire does not address the patient's past experience, such as: Did you suffer from abuse as a child? Did you grow up in a household with your parents or with somebody else? Did your parents attend residential school? In my medical practice with either Indigenous or non-Indigenous patients, I need to establish any background related to childhood trauma, but in an indirect way. To build trust, I've learned to support the patient in volunteering sensitive information. I can ask directly: Do you drink alcohol? How much do you drink? I dutifully record the response in the patient's medical record, and so it is documented. Asking the question Why do you drink? is a heavier business that requires an ongoing relationship. Through my experience with patients like Sylvia, I have become more skilled at respectfully encouraging patients to tell me about the degrees of childhood trauma. The trauma, for example, related to growing up with a troubled family on reserve, or the scarring trauma of being removed from that family. In my view, these traumatic factors are more important than the CAGE criteria.

+ + +

A year after Sylvia's return from the treatment program at Indian Head, she is admitted to the Regina General Hospital again after an assault by her new common-law husband. She arrives by ambulance, complaining of abdominal pain. She had been struck repeatedly in the face and abdomen; she was anemic and received a transfusion of two units of blood. After we move her upstairs, she is referred to a social worker for addiction and spousal-abuse counselling. At the end of her stay, I again give her an appointment for follow-up in my office. This time, she comes and tells me she has stopped drinking. She will be moving to a basement apartment to live by herself. I prescribe vitamins and an antidepressant, and we discuss the benefits of attending Alcoholics Anonymous meetings.

Two weeks later she is back at my office and says she has started to drink again. She asks for another referral to the treatment centre. I fill out the government forms that give her high priority for admission and don't see her again for several months.

Many of Canada's Indigenous communities have tried to reduce the costs related to alcohol use disorder by prohibiting the transportation of alcohol onto reserves. This choice goes back to the beginning of treaty-making; the chiefs who negotiated Treaty 6, for example, requested a ban on alcohol on reserves.[13] The Government of Canada followed up, in 1884, with a general ban on the sale of liquor to Indians under Section 94 of the Indian Act. This was recognized, after many years, as discriminatory, and in 1951 the provinces were given discretion to allow the sale of alcohol to Indians in licensed taverns. However, access remained hit and miss. It was not until 1971 that a Supreme Court of Canada ruling led to the abolition of Section 94.

The federal liquor ban was a major factor in the implementation of the pass system—whereby, until 1941, an Indian agent controlled each Indian coming and going from reserve. This system kept Indigenous adults on reserve while their children were taken away to residential schools. The schools and the teaching of settler ways were a primary tool in Canada's assimilation strategy. The destruction of families led to the loss of traditional connection with the land and the exile of many

---

13   Johnson, *Firewater*.

residential school Survivors into the cities, where they could obtain alcohol. Meanwhile, those who remained on reserve developed links to local homebrew producers. In a political economy that promoted capitalism, bootlegging to the reserve became a source of income.

There are some that believe that the prohibition of alcohol on reserves over many decades contributed to the phenomenon of binge drinking, also called heavy episodic drinking (HED), especially among adolescents. As young people become adults, continued HED creates financial stress. When the welfare cheque comes in, people are more likely to spend it on drink and then go without cash for the rest of the month. As Chief Robert Joseph, an educator and member of the Gwawaenuk First Nation in British Columbia, has noted, "the *Indian Act* prohibition [on alcohol] set the stage for the pervasive stereotype that Indians suffer from alcohol intolerance."[14]

The myth of the drunken Indian was exacerbated by medical literature. In 1971, the *Canadian Medical Association Journal* published a paper entitled "Ethanol Metabolism in Various Racial Groups."[15] In this study, hospitalized Indigenous patients and white hospital staff in Edmonton were infused with alcohol intravenously to achieve a blood level of 125 mg/dl. Using a breathalyzer, researchers then measured the rate of disappearance of the alcohol. The authors conclude that Indigenous people metabolize alcohol at a slower rate than white people and hypothesize that this is due to genetic differences. This result has been quoted many times by the medical profession. The CMAJ article states that the subjects in this study were volunteers but does not mention

---

14   Bob Joseph, "A Look at First Nations Prohibition of Alcohol," Indigenous Corporate Training, October 20, 2016, https://www.ictinc.ca/blog/first-nations-prohibition-of-alcohol.

15   D. Fenna, O. Schaefer, L. Mix, and J.A. Gilbert, "Ethanol Metabolism in Various Racial Groups," *Canadian Medical Association Journal* 105, no. 5 (September 4, 1971): 472–475, https://pubmed.ncbi.nlm.nih.gov/5112118/.

a consent form or ethics review. This example from medical science seems to support the common complaint among Indigenous people—a complaint that many of my patients have presented to me—that settlers have experimented on them and their families.[16]

The 1971 study and others perpetuated the medical myth that Indigenous people were susceptible to alcoholism. However, other studies such as research from the University of Alaska published over twenty years later in 1992[17] have shown this is false. In fact, the Alaska researchers concluded that Indigenous people metabolize alcohol faster than settler people. The myth has been busted, but the prevailing attitude of the settler was cemented into both popular and medical culture. Helpful whites with liberal values continue to insist that the "drunken Indian" problem is one that can be solved by public health messages that educate the public about the dangers of alcohol, without addressing the embedded racism. In fact, the methods proven to solve alcohol dependence in any society are the same as those that address smoking or drug addiction: restricting availability, increasing pricing controls, regulating marketing to young people, and increasing accessibility and funding for treatment programs.

---

16   Brian Schnarch, "Ownership, Control, Access and Possession (OCAP) or Self-Determination Applied to Research: A Critical Analysis of Contemporary First Nations Research and Some Options for First Nations Communities," *Journal of Aboriginal Health* 1, no. 1 (2004), https://jps.library.utoronto.ca/index.php/ijih/article/view/28934.

17   B. Segal and L.K. Duffy, "Ethanol Elimination among Different Racial Groups," *Alcohol* 9, no. 3 (May–June 1992): 213–217, https://doi.org/10.1016/0741-8329(92)90056-g. See also the National Research Council (US) Committee on Population's "Overview of Alcohol Abuse Epidemiology for American Indian Populations" in Gary D. Sandefur, Ronald R. Rindfuss, and Barney Cohen, editors, *Changing Numbers, Changing Needs: American Indian Demography and Public Health* (Washington, DC: National Academies Press, 1996). This report cites a dozen studies: "In general, the findings have shown that American Indians metabolize alcohol in a manner and at a speed similar to those of other ethnic groups in the United States."

As the medical profession debated the interaction between Indigenous identity and alcohol, a new generation of self-empowered Indigenous leaders considered the options for taking action. The federal Royal Commission on Aboriginal Peoples, commissioned in 1991, heard evidence from Indigenous leaders and citizens on racism and abuse in the residential school system, among many other issues. One outcome of the commission's report was the creation of the Aboriginal Healing Foundation (AHF), funded for $350 million (until funding ceased in 2014) to address residential school trauma.

+ + +

In our meeting before she left Regina for her second attempt at rehabilitation, Sylvia revealed important family history. Although her mother was an alcoholic, not all of her childhood was tragic. Her father had served a term as Chief, and her mother was respected for her skill with traditional crafts. Sylvia was surrounded by brothers and sisters during her years living at home, and she attended a nearby day school run by the community administration.[18] She married a man from a reserve near Regina when she was eighteen, and they had two children. She divorced him twice and remarried him twice. One of her daughters lives in Ontario, the other in British Columbia. She was, however, silent about her time in residential school for most of our conversation, until she told me how happy she had been to receive a big cheque from Ottawa, a payment in response to her residential school claim.

Just a few days later, at 11:00 p.m. on a Saturday night, my cellphone rings. I answer it hesitantly. I am not on call, and I am not expecting to

---

18 The British North American (BNA) Act of 1867 delegated jurisdiction for education to the provinces, while the Numbered Treaties protected rights to education for Indigenous Peoples. In 1972, the National Indian Brotherhood (now called Assembly of First Nations) advocated for control of Indigenous education and federal funding allowed for on-reserve day schools.

hear from a patient. It's Sylvia, speaking in a high-pitched, rapid-fire pattern consistent with severe anxiety. I realize that sometime in the past I must have called her from my mobile number without making it anonymous. She is calling me from the ER, breathless and crying. A gang has come to her house and broken her windows. She is afraid to go home.

I get in my car and drive to the hospital Emergency entrance. Sylvia is standing just inside next to a slender, dark-haired man. His name, I learn, is Daniel. I don't know if this is the common-law husband who assaulted her the year before. He has bruises on his face and a long laceration over his scalp that has been stitched up by the ER physician. He appears high. He can't focus his eyes, and after saying hello to me, he wanders away to a vacant gurney where he falls asleep. The ER physician doesn't know what to do with them. Sylvia's anxiety about broken windows at the house does not meet the criteria for admission to hospital. However, I negotiate an overnight stay for the couple. We give her a sleeping pill, and she crawls onto the gurney in the holding area where Daniel is passed out. When I leave for the night, she is nestled spoon-like with him. It occurs to me that Sylvia and Daniel may have some connection with gang life.

In her conversations with me, Sylvia had skated past her experience, or her family's experience, with residential school. This is true for many of my patients, but the intergenerational effects from the schools run deep. These effects are caused by something called observational distress. Through animal studies, scientists have learned that the fear suffered by others leaves a neural trace that predisposes the observer to experience trauma later on. In other words, if a human being watches another person experience stress, their brain is preconditioned to experience stress with very little stimulus.

The amygdala (the emotion and survival centre in the brain) is particularly affected by stress. The prefrontal cortex, the planning and decision-making area, is inhibited when the amygdala is excited. The cortex governs executive functions like planning, self-monitoring, self-control, and time management, all of them important in the Western linear world. These skills are needed to find housing, apply for a job, manage a household, do laundry, buy groceries, and manage a bank account. Without these skills, fitting into the white settler world that surrounds the Indigenous community is difficult and stressful. When an individual is governed by emotion and panic, it's hard for them to recruit the executive functions.

The next morning, I return to the ER holding area. Daniel has gone. Sylvia is alone, dressed and composed, sitting up on the gurney. She's putting on her winter coat as I enter; she glances at me, gives a brave smile, and walks towards the exit. She waves at me as she leaves.

A month later, Sylvia is sitting in my office once again. She reports that her life has taken a turn for the better. Her black hair is carefully done up, with curled tendrils resting around her face. She is wearing jeans and a blouse. She has gone to rehab and met a new man. They are planning to move in together. She has reconnected with her twenty-one-year-old daughter, who has agreed to take care of Sylvia's bank account. Sylvia has won $37,000 in the lottery and bought a car. She has stopped drinking, is eating well, and appears happy. She asks me to refill her prescription for antidepressants, and I comply. Her abdomen is soft, without evidence of fluid accumulation.

She is doing well, for now.

Neither one of us knows that her new-found love is HIV positive.

✛ ✛ ✛

A year later, Sylvia appears again in the waiting area of the Regina General. She looks thin and wasted, except for a large belly that I soon determine is filled with fluid, the sign of a severely damaged liver. Her blood work is troubling, and her lymphocyte count is very low. She has experienced recurrent infections. We order an HIV test, and it comes back positive. Her liver is so damaged that her system will not tolerate the cocktail of HIV drugs that might have saved her. There's nothing more the health system can do—and there's nothing left for me to do but go home and cry.

Sylvia was an attractive, engaging woman who died at age fifty-one of self-inflicted attempts to soothe her personal pain. Over the five years that I knew her, she suffered damage related to intergenerational trauma from residential schools, gang life in Regina, housing problems, addictions, struggles in rehab, and marital abuse. I did my best to make time and space for Sylvia and treat her with respect. I truly believed that if she had been provided with support, she might have beaten her addiction. Naively, perhaps, in my middle-class privileged world, I believed that she could overcome the barriers and get clean.

Beyond providing a bed in hospital on the night that Sylvia fled from her home with broken windows, I don't really know what she hoped I could do for her. Even after my years in the Regina hospital system, a part of me still assumed that my medical training and my institution, with its doctors and nurses and social workers, its pills and machinery, would save her. Like an evangelical preacher, I thought that if she would only believe, she would be saved. But the sad truth is that I could not be with her for the multiple times that her life fell apart. I could never truly understand the tangled effects of the residential school trauma that she and her family had suffered, or the underlying trauma related to the destruction of her people's traditional way of life. She survived for one month after we discovered her HIV status combined with liver cirrhosis. Her obituary in the local paper said that she would be joining her parents in the Spirit World. I think about that Spirit World often and hope her pain is gone.

MAYBE I WILL, MAYBE I WON'T

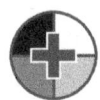

There is little industry on the reserves. Some residents have farms, but most live on small urban-sized plots, in wooden houses or single-wide trailers scattered alongside the roads. The logic of this layout isn't clear to me. In traditional society, the Plains tribes would set up their tipis in a circle or a tight cluster. However, the establishment of the reserve system seems to have destroyed their close-knit pattern of community. If I make more than one home visit on a reserve, I may have to drive for several kilometres from house to house.

There is no centre of town. The band office and the health centre may be located far apart. For most Indigenous people on reserve, nothing is within walking distance. There might be a corner store near the school, or close to the band office, but its prime function is to serve as a cash register for the gas station; the food supply is limited to chips, candy, and sugar-sweetened soda drinks. A lot of people are unemployed. Some work at the band office or the school. One of my patients is the school bus driver, and another is the school janitor, both paid from funds allocated to each reserve from Indigenous Services Canada.

When I take part in clinics on the reserve, my patients talk about the violence in their lives. Domestic abuse and sexual assault are common on the reserve, as well as for Indigenous people in the city. Overall, Indigenous women are almost twice as likely as non-Indigenous women (42 percent as compared to 22 percent, respectively) in their lifetime to experience physical abuse at the hands of an intimate partner.[1] Despair and resignation are rampant, reinforced by white colonialist attitudes in the surrounding rural area. If it were not for the non-Indigenous living conditions imposed upon them, most of the Indigenous people that I see would not have to endure violence, poverty, and food insecurity. The destruction of the Indigenous world view of harmony, cooperation, and connection to the land has effectively diminished the power of spiritual belief.

When people from the reserve travel to the big city, they see wealthy folk going to work in their sleek cars and expensive clothes. They contrast this with the lives of their relatives, who often live in cramped houses in North Central Regina where bitter winds blow through the walls in winter and cockroaches flourish in summer. Many of the children in those city houses go to school hungry. The slum landlord knocks on the front door every month. When the tenants can no longer pay rent, they return to the reserve, where they bunk in with family for weeks or months until they figure out how to get back to the bright lights. In the end, the city offers its own community; the houses are close together, and people who have fled the reserve can find and interact with people who have shared similar experiences.

---

1   Loanna Heidinger, "Intimate Partner Violence: Experiences of First Nations, Métis and Inuit Women in Canada, 2018," Canadian Centre for Justice and Community Safety Statistics, Statistics Canada, May 19, 2021, https://www150.statcan.gc.ca/n1/pub/85-002-x/2021001/article/00007-eng.htm.

Drugs may promise an escape from the cycle of despair or a pathway into a social network. The lives of drug users are of no interest to the mainstream community until the police come by to investigate a robbery or drug deal. If there is an arrest, a sort of story may be reported in the local newspaper, sometimes with subtle, casual racism embedded in the text of the article. Of course, back on the reserve my patients tell me that some white people are not so bad—the people who do good things and show humility. However, in my opinion, too many of these people are unaware of the dangers and instability that are a daily diet for many Indigenous people.

Soon after I started work at Regina General, I developed an interest in the lives of Indigenous patients. I became a full-fledged member of the order of ignorant, self-righteous white do-gooders. Monias, they call us—a reference to white people that originated from the First Nations description of the Métis fur traders in Western Canada, who worked for the Hudson's Bay Company. As the Wellness Wheel project matured, I came to feel more confident in my interactions with Indigenous patients. I learned about life on reserve, and the flow of drugs, money, and people between the reserve and the city. My monias was getting an education from patients like Maureen.

Maureen, a woman from the poorest section of North Central in Regina, comes to the ER with severe back pain and says she can't walk. She is experiencing fevers and chills. Neil, a former medical student whom I taught, is now the ER physician who assesses her, and he decides that she shouldn't go home. By the time I see Maureen—after a change in shifts and a stay overnight while waiting for test results to return—she has been waiting in the ER for eighteen hours and she's curled up in the fetal position on a stretcher. She has a sheet over her head, and I hear only muffled sounds in response to my greeting. I hope she can feel my concerned presence.

"Maureen, I understand you're having back pain. How long has it been going on?"

I see the slight, thin body twitch under the sheet, dishevelled hair at one end, a jean-clad leg sticking out the other. There is a muffled grunt; a small hand appears, pulling the sheet even further over her head. If I push and ask more medical questions, she will distrust me. If I leave, she may talk with me on my next visit. I decide that the best course of action is to give her time and space, since she will not interact with me now. I walk to the main desk and write Maureen's admission orders, including an order for blood cultures. I hope she will stay, and I'm betting that her pain and her inability to walk will encourage her to remain in our care, overriding any desire she may have to avoid suffering through a hospitalization.

It will be best to give her intravenous antibiotics on the assumption that she has an infection in her spine that is affecting her ability to walk. She's been using IV drugs, and her veins are a mess, but one of the nurses manages to get a PICC (peripherally inserted central catheter) inserted into her left arm. I give Maureen hydromorphone, an opioid derivative, for her pain. I strongly suspect an abscess at her spine, and I ask for an MRI scan. At her bedside leaning over the shroud on the gurney, I try to explain what we are doing to help. After my monologue, there's no answer, but I can see the steady rise and fall of the sheet, so I know she is still breathing. The porter arrives to take her upstairs to a private room.

In addition to scanning her spine, we'll do complex screening of her blood samples to check for infection—HIV, Hepatitis C, and sexually transmitted conditions such as syphilis. When I entered medical school, we regarded syphilis as a very rare disease. It had been common in the time of Shakespeare, and in that of Queen Victoria, and many famous people were afflicted prior to the discovery of an effective treatment in the 1940s. It was often called the "Great Pretender" because when left untreated it mimics other diseases. After the adoption of antibiotics in the 1940s, many people assumed syphilis had been conquered.

And then it returned, close to home, in Manitoba and British Columbia, and then in Saskatchewan. One of my colleagues reported cases of blindness in two HIV-positive patients. HIV doesn't cause blindness, so the cases were referred to my colleague Dr. Stu Skinner. He tested for syphilis, and voilà, the result came back positive. Suddenly we were testing every patient with "risk factors"—possible high levels of sexual activity—for syphilis. The results were horrifying.

Syphilis is often asymptomatic, or at least the symptoms are often overlooked at first. The major infection site is the genitalia, and the resulting chancre is generally a painless, singular ulceration, which is unlikely to be noticed inside the vagina or rectum or even on the penis. The chancre lasts three to six weeks and heals regardless of whether the individual receives treatment; however, if the person does not receive treatment, syphilis can progress to the secondary stage. It can be a silent disease, or have diffuse symptoms such as fever, swollen lymph glands, rash, headache, or weight loss. If undetected and untreated, it can progress to tertiary syphilis and infect several organ systems, including the brain, heart, and eyes. The key to effective treatment is early detection, since all syphilis infections can be treated in the early stage with one simple shot of benzathine penicillin G. Very few adults have died from syphilis in Canada in recent years, but with the development of antibiotic resistance in those who are allergic to penicillin, the course of treatment is becoming more complicated and the risk of death is growing. Our major problem in Saskatchewan is when people face barriers in finding health care or are fearful or suspicious of doctors.

The World Health Organization advises that syphilis is especially troublesome for pregnant women: "Untreated syphilis infection in pregnancy can lead to stillbirth, neonatal death and congenital disease (collectively defined as 'congenital syphilis')" and also increases the risk of HIV transmission and acquisition in the mother and the infant ("vertical transmission").² At Regina General we have seen significant numbers of pregnant women who showed no symptoms but delivered babies with congenital abnormalities consistent with syphilis.

When our team encounters a patient who uses drugs, we have to treat the primary health issue with every available resource, but we also have to imagine a long list of potential problems. In Maureen's case, tonight, for now, her blood tests come back negative: no HIV, no Hepatitis C, no syphilis. I am relieved when I check the lab results.

The next day, I find her under the sheet in her hospital bed and tell her the results of her MRI—we have found an abscess at the lower part of her spine. More good news: the previous night's antibiotics and narcotics have helped; she's feeling better, and she's lying on her side, uncurled from the fetal position but turned away from me. The neurosurgery team has confirmed that she doesn't need an operation; we can continue to treat the problem with IV antibiotics. She answers my questions in staccato syllables, speaking to the wall. Even though I can't see her face, I suspect that she is not smiling.

A few days later, there is a transformation. Maureen is sitting up, dressed and composed, using a wheelchair to get around her private room. She is slender, her dark hair pulled back into a ponytail. We are getting to know each other. I have been visiting every day to check her pain level, and she has emerged from under her sheet to become an engaging, attractive forty-five-year-old Indigenous woman. She introduces her husband, Wesley, who sits in a plastic chair beside her bed. He is stocky, square-jawed, with straight dark hair that falls to his shoulders. He wears a T-shirt, revealing multiple tattoos on his arms. With my biased eyes, I have the impression that I would be afraid of

---

2   The Global Health Observatory, "Congenital Syphilis—Number of Reported Cases," World Health Organization, https://www.who.int/data/gho/indicator-metadata-registry/imr-details/4492.

him if I were to meet him on the street. Although he appears docile in the sterile hospital room, his eyes are large and black, and glazed. I recognize this docility; he is stoned. During my medical conversation with Maureen, I notice that she glances at him after every answer.

"How are you doing today?" I ask.

"Fine." Glance at Wesley.

"Are you in pain?"

"No, the painkillers are working fine." Glance at Wesley.

"Well, I'm glad to meet your husband."

She smiles at me and then looks at him.

I leave the room with the sinking feeling that she is an abused woman. In her fawning attitude, I interpret subservience and eagerness to please. I suspect there is a codependent relationship, with one drug habit feeding the other.

On my visit the next day, while she is alone in the hospital room, I ask if her husband is going to visit. She confesses to me that he has told her that he wants to leave her because she's always doing drugs. This is the first time that she has mentioned her habit. I had not mentioned drugs previously, although I assumed that her spinal abscess is from infection related to intravenous drugs; it's a common complication among people who use drugs who land in hospital. The needles she has been putting into her arm have been contaminated. As the bacteria float around in her bloodstream, they look for a place to settle. The lower spine is a quiet, unassuming hiding place. It will take a long course of antibiotics to eradicate this nest, but at least Maureen is now able to get out of bed and appears to be improving. She says she wants to quit IV drugs. With tears in her eyes, she says that her children are in custody with her elder sister on reserve—one of the Wellness Wheel reserves.

She is clearly attached to her husband, wants to be healthy, wants to address her addiction, and wants to get her children back. I suspect that there are other circumstances in her background that have prevented her from getting clean. I sign up for a one-day addictions course for health professionals; I am struggling to find the best way to treat Maureen and others like her.

My takeaway from the course is a new insight into a style of addictions treatment called *trauma-informed care*. Technically defined as "practices that promote a culture of safety, empowerment, and healing,"[3] trauma-informed care is taught with the aim to help people find meaning and purpose in their lives, fulfill valued roles, help them pursue avenues to reduce distress and problems, and exercise personal autonomy and self-determination in making choices. The challenge for me, in applying this academic formula, will be to address the multiple traumas that Indigenous people in Canada have endured. It will take a combination of building trust by avoiding the use of triggering language, approaching the patient with sensitivity, and using non-threatening body language.

I'm reminded in the workshop that addictions are often associated with adverse childhood experiences (ACE). A foundational study of ACE in 1998[4] presented a long list of such experiences: physical abuse, sexual abuse, emotional abuse, physical neglect, emotional neglect, violence against a mother, parental divorce, household member having problems with substances, household member having problems with mental illness, and incarceration of a household member. This aligns

---

3   Monique Tello, "Trauma-Informed Care: What It Is and Why It's Important," Harvard Health Blog, October 16, 2018, https://www.health.harvard.edu/blog/trauma-informed-care-what-it-is-and-why-its-important-2018101613562.

4   V.J. Felitti, R.F. Anda, D. Nordenberg, D.F. Williamson, A.M. Spitz, V. Edwards, M.P. Koss, and J.S. Marks, "Relationship of Childhood Abuse and Household Dysfunction to Many of the Leading Causes of Death in Adults. The Adverse Childhood Experiences (ACE) Study," *American Journal of Preventitive Medicine* 14, no. 4 (May 1998): 245–258, https://doi.org/10.1016/s0749-3797(98)00017-8.

with my own experience, based on interviews with patients who have addictions or live with addiction in their families. I learned that there is a dose response to trauma; the more severe the adverse experiences, the more likely that someone will develop a maladaptive coping mechanism. They are also more likely to have health problems.

Trauma is often present even if patients don't talk about it. It is pervasive. Maureen, during one of our visits, confesses that she was abandoned by her mother at an early age, and she doesn't want to be abandoned by her husband. This, despite the fact that her husband, I suspect, is taking drugs, providing them to her, and then reacting in outrage when she takes them.

I have hopes for Maureen's recovery from drug addiction, but I also have to abide by the hospital rules. If a patient has a stable household and no relationship with street drugs, we show them how to hook up their medications to a PICC line and infuse their daily dose at home. Maureen's case, however, sends up some red flags. I sit down on the side of her bed and explain that because she's a person who uses drugs, the rules will not allow her to use a PICC regimen at her home in north Regina. There's a risk that she would use the equipment to get high in an environment where there are abundant street drugs. If she wants to get well, she has to agree to six weeks of hospitalization.

She asks if she can go back to reserve and manage her treatment with her elder sister and children close by.

I ask: "Will you be safe on reserve?"

She says: "My community is there to support me, and I want to be clean."

Through Wellness Wheel, I have a relationship with the home care nurse on the reserve where Maureen grew up and where her elder sister lives. I call the home care nurse at one of the Touchwood Hills clinics and explain the situation. The safest place for Maureen—if she insists on leaving the hospital—is with her sister, not in the city with a controlling husband. The home care nurse on reserve spoke with the sister, who says she will take responsibility for accepting Maureen back onto the reserve and for protecting her from the dangers of the city.

We get the necessary permission from hospital management. I meet with one of the hospital's social workers to design a safe home regimen, and we look at how it can be tailored for life on the reserve. I make arrangements with the pharmacy to have antibiotics delivered to the reserve. After hours of phone calls and discussions, we are set. I return to Maureen's room to describe the plan. Will she be okay with it? She appreciates the time that I have spent to help her, and she's relieved that she won't have to stay in hospital for six weeks.

As I make my rounds on the medical ward later that day, I bump into the social worker, a colleague of mine named Paula, who stops me in the corridor. She is wearing tall boots and looks imposing, although her demeanour is warm and empathetic. She cares about the patients she interacts with. We both want to avoid sending a person who has a history of using drugs into an unsafe environment. She has just spoken with Maureen.

"She told me that you agreed to send her home to be with her husband in Regina during her course of IV antibiotics," Paula states matter-of-factly.

I feel dismay. I have spent hours of my time making phone calls to arrange a special treatment program for her, using ingenuity and advocacy for my patient. I'm having the kind of emotional reaction that doctors are not supposed to have, and I recognize that this reaction could turn into anger towards the patient. After the work that I have done, and the daily visits to prepare her for the return to the reserve, why would Maureen tell this story to Paula? Does she really believe that we will break the rules so she can put herself at risk?

Splitting and triangulation happen when children go to one parent to ask permission, then go to the other parent when the first says no.

After cooling down for a couple of hours, I ask Paula to accompany me to Maureen's room. I sit on the side of Maureen's bed. Paula sits on the plastic chair in the corner.

I ask Maureen an open-ended question without judgment: "What's your understanding of our plan for discharge?"

She looks me in the eye and tells me that she is going to the reserve to be with her sister and receive six weeks of antibiotics.

Paula speaks up now. "Why did you tell me something different?"

Maureen replies, "I didn't know who you were. You just came into my room and started asking questions."

I look at Maureen. "Why did you lie?"

She responds: "Because I'm good at it. I learned from an early age that I can lie and get away with it. It's easy for me to fool people. I'm good at it."

I am taken aback by her frankness. With Paula in the room, and me sitting on the side of the bed, and Maureen nicely groomed in the bed, we review the plan for treatment on reserve. The timetable is set, the *t*'s crossed, the *i*'s dotted. The strong relationship we have with Maureen's home community and the home care nurse on reserve reassures me that we have a safe plan. Maureen agrees, again, to stay with her sister and reunite with her kids. We will wait for Maureen's sister to get a ride into Regina to pick up Maureen.

Once again, the plan falls apart. Maureen's sister arrives, but she is admitted to hospital with chest pain. Maureen goes for a smoke break outside the hospital and scores some drugs. She gets high. She wanders back into the hospital in a disoriented state, and a nurse must guide her to her room. With no more options left, we arrange for Maureen to spend six weeks with us hooked up to the IV antibiotics that are intended to cure the abscess on her spine. After that, she will return to her home in North Central Regina.

I imagine that Maureen and Wesley have continued in their joint drug addiction, if they are still alive. One or both of them may have contracted HIV, Hepatitis C, or syphilis. And it's very possible that they may have come across a bad batch of fentanyl. Even if Maureen went looking for a way to break free from drugs, there is a shortage of addictions treatment programs in Canada, especially for Indigenous people and especially in Saskatchewan.

Trying to provide care to codependent addicts, Indigenous or otherwise, is one of the most challenging parts of a health care professional's job. We walk the line between helping our patients and yielding all control to a destructive disease. Maureen, with her suspected adverse childhood experiences and her exposure to trauma going back generations, had become a resilient master at manipulation. For her, lying had become a mechanism that allowed her to survive—until, because of her addiction, it led her away from survival.

With the passage of years working in a general hospital, I also have learned my own kind of resilience. My self-righteous liberalism and gullibility have been tested; I am better now at enduring unpleasant surprises without taking them personally, while still managing to give a damn. As expressed in the quote often attributed to eighteenth-century Irish writer Oliver Goldsmith: "Success consists of getting up just one more time than you fall."

SWEETGRASS AND CEREMONY

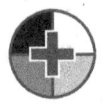

One Christmas Day in Regina, the sky is blue and it is minus twenty degrees Celsius. The streets are quiet. Inside the hospital, every patient who was able to go home has been discharged. I am visiting those who stayed behind on the medical ward, too sick to be sent home. They will receive a Christmas dinner from the hospital cafeteria. The nurses have brought a potluck lunch for themselves, with Crock-Pots and casseroles to share in their break room at the back of the ward. We're all in a good mood.

I am called to the ER at noon. Even here there is a sense of joy, almost a party atmosphere. The ER is quiet. Most patients stay home with their headaches and bandaged thumbs. They are taking the day off. Only the extremely sick come to the ER on Christmas Day.

John, the ER physician, stops me. "There's a young man in room twenty-two with asthma. We've given him nebs, and his breathing has improved. He'll need follow-up. Can you see him before we send him home?"

I enter room twenty-two and find a young, athletic-looking man sitting tall and proud on the edge of the bed. On his fingertip there's an oxygen monitor that is hooked up to a screen. His oxygen saturation shows 85 percent, an acceptable range—likely due to the nebulized bronchodilator therapy, or medicated mist, he's been given to improve his respiration—but still well below normal. However, I know that if he gets up to walk, that level will fall, and he'll feel short of breath. He won't get far.

"Hi! I'm Dr. Boan. I understand you're having trouble breathing."

"My wife and I are driving from our reserve to visit her family in Touchwood Hills. It started in the car, my breathing issue. I haven't had this for a long time. At first I thought it was anxiety, but it kept getting worse."

Jason is twenty-eight years old. There is no audible wheezing when he talks. He looks healthy enough; you wouldn't think there was a problem if it weren't for the numbers on the screen.

"When did you have these symptoms before?" I ask.

"I had asthma when I was a kid. They put me in the hospital. I went to a residential school, and the teachers kept me inside all winter. When I got older, I thought it was related to anxiety, so I went to a traditional healer on the reserve. My asthma got better, but I still have problems. Especially when I'm stressed."

A traditional healer on the reserve. My knowledge of traditional healing is indirect, based on books and college courses in anthropology, with their facts and distortions related to the shaman in traditional cultures. From what I understood, natural healers synthesized the physical and spiritual aspects of the local culture. Traditional healers used local medicinal plants and led their people in healing ceremonies. Wade Davis, an anthropologist from the University of British Columbia, says "the traditional healer bears witness to what is unfolding using ancient wisdom."[1] It is possible that healing and unity—the traditional values

---

1   Wade Davis, "Saving the Planet Means Listening to Indigenous Peoples: Wade Davis," CBC Radio, February 18, 2020, https://www.cbc.ca/radio/ideas/saving-the-planet-means-listening-to-indigenous-peoples-wade-davis-1.5467071.

among Indigenous Peoples in Western Canada—went underground due to the imposition of the Indian Act, property allotments, and the attitude of the churches. Yet, Jason has found a traditional healer on reserve.

Among the multiple texts I consulted while I attended university, I don't remember if any of them dealt with traditions of unity and Indigenous spiritual beliefs, so I don't know what Jason has experienced with his traditional healer—but he appears to believe that it helped him. For now, however, I can only use Western allopathic medicine to help his breathing.

I pull my stethoscope from the pocket of my white coat and move closer to the bedside. "I am going to listen now; just breathe normally." Now I hear the wheezing: a high-pitched, musical sound amplified by my stethoscope. Asthma has been described by people who live with it as the feeling of breathing through a straw. The smooth muscles lining our airways can go into spasm for a variety of reasons, and it becomes more difficult to move air in and out of the lungs. Few sensations are as frightening as not being able to get enough air. The sensation of limited airflow can produce anxiety, since the receptors in the chest wall, chemoreceptors, and pulmonary vagal receptors activate brainstem respiratory neurons in the brain.[2]

So is it the anxiety that is driving the asthma, or the asthma that's driving the anxiety? If we're lucky, we'll have Jason and his family on their way before we need to figure this out. Another patient of mine told me that he could feel a shortness of breath before he even realized that it had been triggered by a memory from his past. Jason may be especially vulnerable at Christmas—Was he allowed to leave the residential school to go home? Was there trauma in the home during the

---

2   Francesco Gigliotti, "Mechanisms of Dyspnea in Healthy Subjects," *Multidisciplinary Respiratory Medicine* 5, no. 3 (2010): 195–201, https://doi.org/10.1186/2049-6958-5-3-195.

holiday? This is not the time to ask. I'm just grateful that he is perfectly calm, making the best of this unwanted pit stop.

Jason tells me he has three kids in the car outside waiting with his wife, and a trunk-load of Christmas presents and winter clothes. They need to get to the Touchwood Hills by the end of the day. After another nebulizer treatment, his lungs open up and his oxygen level improves. I prescribe an inhaler, suggest that he avoid rooms with cigarette smoke, and invite him to return to hospital if his breathing does not improve. I'm confident that he will be okay this Christmas.

The fact that he went to a traditional healer for his asthma makes sense to me. I have learned that the natural reaction of most Indigenous people is to first ask for help from a traditional healer on reserve. He had made the connection that his asthma worsened when he was stressed. Inflammation is a prominent feature of asthma, and inflammation is associated with stress. A recent study showed that people with PTSD (post-traumatic stress disorder) have double the risk of developing asthma, especially if they are under the age of twenty.[3] Many studies have linked residential school attendance to post-traumatic stress reactions that can last a lifetime. Jason showed resilience in seeking the services of a traditional healer to resolve his medical condition. Like many of my patients, he did not talk to me about the stress associated with residential school. He just told me that by using traditional healing, his symptoms improved. It may be that, like trauma, resilience is epigenetic—that is, it may be inherited—but the science behind this finding is preliminary.[4]

---

3   Yi-Hsuan Hung, Chih-Ming Cheng, Wei-Chen Lin, Ya-Mei Bai, Tung-Ping Su, Cheng-Ta Li, Shih-Jen Tsai, Tai-Long Pan, Tzeng-Ji Chen, and Mu-Hong Chen, "Post-Traumatic Stress Disorder and Asthma Risk: A Nationwide Longitudinal Study," *Psychiatry Research* 276 (2019): 25–30. https://doi.org/10.1016/j.psychres.2019.04.014.

4   Mary Annette Pember, "Trauma May Be Woven in DNA of Native Americans," *Indian Country Today* (May 28, 2015).

After the training day on addictions when I learned about the concept of trauma-informed care, I began to notice it fitting into my medical practice on a recurring basis. I meet so many Indigenous people who have experienced trauma directly or absorbed it from their parents and grandparents. Anybody with lack of control over their financial and physical circumstances will experience stress. Childhood trauma and recognizing the stress that is associated with it results in an ability to be attuned to subtle reactions from those around you. Sometimes it is the dismissive attitude in the care provider. Other times it can be the minimizing of the symptoms. Worst of all is the contempt that flickers across the face of the health care provider. The sensitivity to detect inauthentic mannerisms is highly developed in people who have experienced trauma. I have noted inauthentic mannerisms of doctors, nurses, and social workers who smile at Indigenous patients and move on. If the recipient of these actions is brave enough to articulate what they're thinking, they might say: "You don't really understand me. You're just pretending."

I was clearly unable to offer Jason support from a place of natural healing, but I did make the effort to connect with him in a natural and authentic way. Trauma-informed care focuses on providing a safe and welcoming experience, a transparent and consistent account of what the patient can expect, and a sharing of control.

My Christmas Day meeting with Jason led me to look further into the healing practices of the Indigenous Peoples of Saskatchewan. Central to the traditional approach is the Medicine Wheel concept, balancing the four elements of physical, emotional, mental, and spiritual health, the ways of knowing and being. Several traditional plants—sweetgrass, for example—are used ceremonially to further the holistic approach.

Wade Davis, who studies Indigenous cultures worldwide, spoke on CBC Radio's *Ideas* about the value of ancient wisdom. Davis proposes that we need to make the world safe for cultural differences that include the Indigenous perspective. In particular, he stressed that in Indigenous teachings it is our relationships that become the medicine[5]—that is, our relationships with the earth, plants, animals, each other, and the cosmos. All of these relationships are interconnected and encompassing. This is the meaning of the Cree term wâhkôhtowin, which refers to our relationships with all things.

Many Canadians, including Indigenous people, practise medical pluralism, trying to choose the best treatments from more than one medical system. Over one-third of all Canadians visit alternative health practitioners—such as physical therapists, acupuncturists, homeopaths, naturopaths, and holistic healers. The physician is seen as someone who alleviates symptoms, while a healer eliminates the cause of the illness. The patient may choose to stay away from the physician until their symptoms are severe. With most of the alternative systems the patient maintains more control, and with traditional medicine the treatment is generally, but not always, less expensive than the white man's pills. The risk, obviously, is that the patient may bypass an innovative cure offered in the Western medicine realm and suffer fatal consequences.

Indigenous healing is based on the traditions that are kept by the Elders in the community, the Knowledge Keepers. As I learn more about Indigenous people in Saskatchewan, I discover that Knowledge Keepers are more than librarians who keep facts in a repository for people to access, or a history buff who knows the dates of the treaty signing. Traditional values are linked in a circle—the land, the spirits, the ancestors. Traditional medicine thought patterns are nonlinear, circular, as they access the supernatural.

---

5   Davis, "Saving the Planet Means Listening to Indigenous Peoples."

The Medicine Wheel is a universal symbol of cosmic unity,[6] the circle of life that encompasses the earth's cycles of renewal, the changing seasons, the sun, the stars, and humanity's relationship with the earth and the cosmos. As I explored Indigenous spirituality and healing practices, I discovered the four quadrants—physical, mental, emotional, and spiritual—connected with a holistic approach, both integrated and interdependent. It has been suggested by some scholars that the Medicine Wheel is an example of cultural appropriation, as a way of organizing complex culture knowledge into four parts, not previously described by Indigenous culture.[7] A revision of the Medicine Wheel adds a centre circle referred to as holism, balance, and harmony.[8] I was beginning to see the Medicine Wheel as a symbol to explain a complex interconnectedness with nature, life cycles, weather, spirituality, and culture. As explained by Lloyd Hawkeye Robertson:

> I taught an undergraduate university class on contemporary native health issues in which students were invited to create their own personal medicine wheel. While many drew a wheel with four divisions, the number of spokes ranged from 0 to 18. One aboriginal person drew a series of concentric circles with herself surrounded by family, community, "helpers" (meaning outside agencies such as educators and counselors), and "white" society. Another student used spokes to

---

[6] Robert Regnier, "The Sacred Circle: A Process Pedagogy of Healing," *Interchange* 25, no. 2 (1994): 129–144, https://link.springer.com/content/pdf/10.1007/BF01534540.pdf.

[7] Robertson, "The Medicine Wheel Revisited"; Frances Widdowson and Albert Howard, "Running the Gauntlet: Challenging the Taboo Obstructing Aboriginal Education Policy Development," in ed. Widdowson and Howard, *Approaches to Aboriginal Education in Canada: Searching for Solutions* (Calgary: Brush Education, 2013), 288–317.

[8] Richard L. Roberts, Ruth Harper, Donna Tuttle-Eagle Bull, Lynn M. Heideman-Provost, "The Native American Medicine Wheel and Individual Psychology: Common Themes," *The Journal of Individual Psychology* 54, no. 1 (1998): 135–146.

divide a circle into categories representing vision, compassion, family, work, education, language (Cree), planning, doing, love, nature, and God. Although it might be possible to reduce such a self-characterization to four more general categories, doing so serves to constrain the individual's meaning and relational experience.[9]

Several days after meeting Jason in the ER, I decided to go to my local church. The speaker giving the sermon was an astronomer who worked at the local university. Her sermon explored the reality that we, as settlers, live in the third dimension of our reality—the length, width, and depth of all objects in our universe. Then she began to explore the other dimensions that we may not be perceiving beyond our visible dimensions. She mentions the fourth dimension—time; the knowledge of an object's position in time is essential to plotting its position in the universe. I believe Einstein received a Nobel Prize for explaining the theory of relativity to the Western world. Then she becomes philosophical about our perceptions of our reality. She begins to explore the fifth and sixth dimensions. She says, "If we could see on through to the fifth dimension, we would see a world slightly different from our own, giving us a means of measuring the similarity and differences between our world and other possible ones." Then she explores the sixth dimension—the concept that most things in life are limited by our own perception of what we know and don't know as well as our understanding of past and current events in our lives. The sixth dimension is a higher level of existence that exists outside time and imagination and lies somewhere between truth and that which should never be seen. I realized that spirituality was supernatural, holistic, and unseen. Healing was connected to the supernatural if I could integrate the dimensions.

---

9   Robertson, "The Medicine Wheel Revisited."

By the time I stumble out of the church, my reality has been changed. Indigenous ancestors knew about different dimensions, but I was only taught about three in my white settler reality. Well, maybe four—I understand the concept of time—but I had no idea about the fifth or sixth dimensions of reality. In a time when there were no clocks or calendars, the people looked to the stars, the planets, the sun, and the weather to predict the time—present, past, and future—and the interconnectedness of all life.

With my new-found perspective, I began to see the Medicine Wheel as a sphere that links modern allopathic concepts with a deeper supernatural reality. It should be noted that the term *medicine* in Indigenous beliefs often refers to magic or the supernatural—more connected to the supernatural than healing. Every health clinic that I have visited in Saskatchewan has a Medicine Wheel symbol on its wall, which reminds me of the things that I do not know.

I have experienced several ways that traditional medicine interacts with my allopathic, linear views. The use of traditional prairie plants has undergone a revival in smudging, purification at the Sweat Lodge, and sacred singing and dancing. Sweetgrass plays a prominent part in traditional healing ceremonies. It is a wild plant native to the North American prairies, harvested and braided. As it burns, it has a sweet scent, and its smoke is believed to purify thoughts and prevent negative thinking. It is used in talking circles and smudges. Prairie sage, with a stronger scent than sweetgrass, is used to purify mind, body, and spirit. It is believed that it creates a barrier to prevent evil spirits from entering a room before a ceremony. Scientific analysis of sage has shown it to have antifungal, antiseptic, and astringent properties and to be high in polyphenols, which are thought to be biochemical scavengers that negate free radicals by forming stabilized chemical complexes that lead to protective effects against many inflammation-mediated chronic diseases.

Smudging often involves burning traditional herbal plants in a bowl or abalone shell and wafting the smoke around the area that requires purification. I have seen this ceremony often at gatherings, where the hands are cupped over the bowl and the smoke pulled up over the head. When I first saw it performed, I assumed that the head needed healing. Then I realized that the act of wafting smoke around your head was supposed to purify the thoughts. Despite the lack of scientific evidence that sweetgrass and sage will produce molecular changes to the brain by gently wafting smoke around the head, the ceremony is surprisingly peaceful and centering.

Tobacco is another traditional medicine that I have learned about. Wild tobacco was used long before contact with Europeans, dating back at least 1,100 years.[10] Through hybridization of tobacco found in the Peruvian Andes by early explorers, *Nicotiana tabacum* has become the domesticated marketed form of tobacco.[11] The wild tobacco found in the Great Plains, *Nicotiana attenuata*, was used for gifts, prayers, offerings, and ceremonies. The active ingredient in tobacco, nicotine, is known to decrease heart rate, alter consciousness, and in high doses can induce a catatonic state. These effects made the use of tobacco important in ceremonial or religious rituals, and its use took on a supernatural and sacred quality among Indigenous people.

Because of its use in ceremonies, the federal government imposed policies to inhibit the ceremonial use of tobacco by Indigenous people.

---

10   Shannon Tushingham and Jelmer W. Eerkens, "Hunter-Gatherer Tobacco Smoking in Ancient North America: Current Chemical Evidence and a Framework for Future Studies," in *Perspectives on the Archaeology of Pipes, Tobacco and other Smoke Plants in the Ancient Americas*, eds. Elizabeth A. Bollwerk and Shannon Tushingham (Springer, Cham.: Interdisciplinary Contributions to Archaeology, 2016), 211–230, https://doi.org/10.1007/978-3-319-23552-3_12.

11   Tonio Sadik, "Traditional Use of Tobacco among Indigenous Peoples in North America," March 28, 2014, https://cottfn.com/wp-content/uploads/2015/11/TUT-Literature-Review.pdf.

In addition to banning Indigenous dances, ceremonies, and festivals, an Indian Act amendment in 1895 prohibited the selling of produce from Indian reserves in an effort to kill Indigenous ceremonial traditions. Meanwhile, the domestication of tobacco resulted in a worldwide push to promote its use by tobacco companies. Cigarette smoking reached its peak in North America in the 1950s when smoking was thought to be glamorous, and it was not until 1964 that smoking was scientifically proven to be harmful.

To understand the degree to which the tobacco companies invested in scientific explorations of the addictive nature of nicotine is to recognize the colonial agenda of promoting cigarette smoking in Indigenous communities. Red Man chewing tobacco, first marketed in 1904, only removed its iconic American Indian logo in 2022. In the 1980s, R.J. Reynolds Company began marketing Natural American Spirit cigarettes with the symbol of an American Indian in a headdress holding a ceremonial pipe, blurring the distinction between commercial daily use and traditional ceremonial use of tobacco. Additionally, it led to many Indigenous people thinking that Natural American Spirit cigarettes were owned by an Indigenous company and that their profits benefit Indigenous Peoples.[12]

Smoking has become a common addiction among Indigenous people, just as it is among settler populations. Cigarette smoking rates on First Nations reserves are now the highest in Canada, and COPD (chronic obstructive pulmonary disease) is one of the most common diseases on reserves. Smoking cessation programs need to recognize the ceremonial significance of tobacco and separate public health messages about

---

12   Jennifer B. Unger, Claradina Soto, and Lourdes Baezconde-Garbanati, "Perceptions of Ceremonial and Nonceremonial Uses of Tobacco by American-Indian Adolescents in California," *Journal of Adolescent Health* 38, no. 4 (2006): 443, e9–16, https://doi.org/10.1016/j.jadohealth.2005.02.002.

it from its ceremonial use. Despite the known health risks associated with smoking cigarettes, we often take a package of leaf tobacco as a gift to Elders on reserve.

My view of Indigenous cultural practices and healing has grown more complex, year after year, as I learn about them. Every day that I am in a clinic on reserve and interact with Indigenous patients, I learn something new. Although my role is to listen to difficult symptoms, come up with a diagnosis, treat illness, and provide emotional support, I have become acutely aware of the integration of other dimensions in how we approach disease.

I continue to question the values that I was taught as a privileged white person. I was told from birth that I was valuable and through privilege was given advantages to succeed. I was never made to submit to a colonizing power. As a physician, I am part of the decision-making class, at least at a local level. I have been taught that amassing personal wealth and having respect for other people's possessions are integral to our society. While family and friends are important, I was taught that one's personal achievements define one's position in our world. As I move into discovering the fifth dimension, where the world is defined by openness rather than separation, I begin to understand the concept that most things in life are limited by our own perception of what we know and don't know. Through the awakening of at least some aspects of spiritual understanding after my return to Saskatchewan, I have started to explore a different way of seeing. I began to understand that personal relationships are more important than material wealth.

Since the signing of the treaties, government-run child welfare agencies in Canada practised the ongoing removal of Indigenous children from their homes, based on conventional measures of poverty or abuse. Through Section 88 (1951) of the Indian Act, provincial governments were authorized to enforce provincial standards under the Child and Family Services Act. Children were "scooped," generally placed with white families, and are still living among us—as are some of their birth parents, who were often Survivors of residential schools. In 2019, the federal government passed Bill C-92, legislation to enshrine control for First Nations over their own child welfare system. I rejoiced in July 2021 when Cowessess First Nation achieved a landmark negotiated agreement with the federal and provincial governments to reclaim jurisdiction over child welfare. The first of its kind in Canada.[13] As I listened to my patients who had been "scooped," I realized that in my own life I had advantages in resolving my own issues. Hearing their stories of pain wakes up the suppressed pain in my own heart. My challenge as a professional is to focus on empathy for my patients when I am with them, to shift focus from myself to them. I am in the position of healer, white coat over my street clothes and stethoscope around my neck. I am called to help others. I am told, in fact, that the adversity that I have experienced has helped to make me a resourceful person.

In moments of reflection, I think about resilience. What makes one resilient? It is defined as an individual's ability to properly adapt to stress and adversity. It is also the ability to bounce back from stress with a competent response. American developmental psychologist Emmy Werner studied resilience in the 1970s.[14] She looked at a cohort of children who grew up in households where the parents were unemployed, alcoholic, mentally ill, and poor. In their later years, two-thirds of these children exhibited destructive behaviours and experienced chronic unemployment, substance abuse, and teenage pregnancies. One-third did not. What made this one-third more functional? Looking into resilience theory, we find that coping is a process. There are three

---

13   Dan Jones, "Cowessess Takes Control Over Child Welfare," MBC Radio, July 6, 2021, https://www.mbcradio.com/2021/07/cowessess-takes-control-over-child-welfare?msclkid=ccob119dc4b111ec9a72ed4f607aa10a.
14   Emmy E. Werner, "Resilience in Development," *Association for Psychological Science* 4, no. 3 (1995), 81–84, https://doi.org/10.1111/1467-8721.ep10772327.

approaches to a stressful situation: anger, other overwhelming negative emotions, or concern with the disruptive state. The first two reactions lead people to assume the victim role and reject help. The third type of reaction brings about a change in the pattern of disruption and creates a space where the individual develops a coping strategy. In other words, the disruption caused by the trauma is so disturbing that the individual seeks a plan to resolve the disruption. This third type of reaction is called *resilience*.

The twenty-first century has seen a collective uprising of resilience among Canada's Indigenous people. The Truth and Reconciliation Commission of Canada found that the pattern of colonial rule in previous centuries amounted to cultural genocide. But on today's reserves, and in urban classrooms and community halls, traditional ways are in recovery. Organizations offer workshops and training programs that help individuals and communities move forward from the legacy of residential schools. Community resilience requires an integral whole-systems approach that fosters compassion, inner resilience (healthy, respectful, caring relationships), and outer resilience (fair, sustainable sharing systems) within an eco-social region.

Ultimately, I have come to believe that integrating Western medicine with traditional healing methods would offer important benefits to both Indigenous and non-Indigenous people, and it may be essential to the long-term viability of our communities. Meanwhile, despite the nineteenth-century promise of the medicine chest for Indigenous people, our governments are still leaving all Canadians, Indigenous and non-Indigenous, without an optimal health system. I reflect on my learning of the Medicine Wheel and an integrated holistic approach that incorporates things that I may not know, and I am learning to live "in treaty." I continue to learn about traditional medicine and spirituality. In that sense, we are all treaty people.

THE DIALYSIS SHUTTLE

I'm standing in line at the coffee shop near the front door of the hospital, waiting for my morning java fix. I glance over as the door slides open, and I notice a medical van sitting outside with a feather and healing circle logo on the white side panel. A group of patients has arrived from one of the reserves for dialysis. They emerge from the van: One is blind and uses a cane. Another is an amputee in a wheelchair. One is pale, with a yellowish look. All of them have diabetes, and all of them have suffered kidney failure.

When I started working at Regina General, I noticed that the majority of people in the hospital's dialysis room have Indigenous backgrounds. Each patient comes in two or three times a week to sit in a chair hooked up to a machine that cleans their blood. This procedure will extend the life of someone whose kidneys have failed, although not forever; for a fifty-year-old diabetic on dialysis, there is a three in four chance that they will die within ten years.[1]

---

1 Ontario Renal Network, "Discussing Prognosis with Patients on Dialysis: Resource for Healthcare Providers," 2017, https://www.ontariorenalnetwork.ca/sites/renalnetwork/files/assets/discussingprognosis.pdf.

The patients banter with each other and with the nurses. They have accepted that the two or three visits per week to the dialysis room is their life pattern until their heart stops or they receive a kidney transplant.

Among Indigenous people in Saskatchewan, the rate of diabetes, or at least diabetes diagnosis, doubled between 1980 and 1990.[2] By a 2018 estimate, Indigenous people in the province are now three to five times as likely to develop diabetes as the general population.[3] Even worse, the mortality rate for Indigenous people with diabetes is two to three times the rate in the general population.[4] Scientific studies suggest that the high rate of diabetes has a strong genetic cause in Indigenous people, amplified by their position at the social margins—often living in poverty, with limited access to medical care, good food, or recreation.

Kidney failure is just one common risk; many diabetics will develop hypertension or heart disease or require amputations.[5] People with diabetes also have a high prevalence of retinopathy (eye disease) and blindness.

---

2   M. Pioro, R.F. Dyck, and D.C. Gillis. "Diabetes Prevalence Rates Among First Nations Adults on Saskatchewan Reserves in 1990: Comparison by Trail Grouping, Geography and with Non-First Nations People," *Canadian Journal of Pubic Health* 87, no. 5 (1996): 325–328, https://pubmed.ncbi.nlm.nih.gov/8972968/.
3   Brie Hnetka, Diabetes Canada (Saskatchewan), quoted in Cami Kepke, "Sask. Program Mixes Indigenous Culture and Living with Diabetes," Global News, September 27, 2018, https://globalnews.ca/news/4494318/sask-program-mixes-indigenous-culture-and-living-with-diabetes/.
4   Richard T. Oster, Jeffrey A. Johnson, Brenda R. Hemmelgarn, Malcolm King, Stephanie U. Balko, Lawrence W. Svenson, Lindsay Crowshoe, and Ellen L. Toth, "Recent Epidemiologic Trends of Diabetes Mellitus among Status Aboriginal Adults," *Canadian Medical Association Journal* 183, no. 12 (September 6, 2011): E803–E808; Teresa Janz, Joyce Seto, and Annie Turner, "Aboriginal Peoples Survey 2006: An Overview of the Health of the Metis Population," Statistics Canada, 2009, https://www150.statcan.gc.ca/n1/en/catalogue/89-637-X2009004.
5   First Nations and Inuit Regional Health Survey National Steering Committee, "First Nations and Inuit Regional Health Survey," Final Report, 1999, https://fnigc.ca/wp-content/uploads/2020/09/rhs_1997_final_report.pdf.

The high mortality rate for Indigenous diabetics can in part be linked to their lack of access to medical care, but many Indigenous people succeed in finding a doctor: a report from the Regina public health services in 2000 showed that the proportion of local Indigenous people who received medical care from physicians far surpassed the proportion from the general population.[6] However, even with many finding care, many others are living in need. Access to care is extremely difficult for remote populations. Stationing diabetes educators on reserves is a first step, but there are wait times for specialist medical care, and the trip to see a doctor may be a long one. The Saskatchewan government eliminated its government-funded rural bus service in 2017, and many Indigenous people do not own cars. The Government of Canada has stepped in with medical vans to serve the reserves in southern Saskatchewan. People travel to the city in the morning and return at night, and the van is often full. Dialysis treatment is one of the most common uses for the van.

Diabetes is associated with a breakdown of many parts of the body. High blood sugar bathes the internal organs in acid and is especially deleterious for the small blood vessels and kidneys. For Indigenous people, the risk of renal failure and dependence on dialysis is two to three times that in the general population.[7] Moreover, diabetics are at high risk for developing foot ulcers and infections. Untreated foot infections result in destruction of the underlying bone, often necessitating amputations.

---

6   Regina Health District, "Aboriginal Profile—Regina Health District: A Report for Public Health Services, Regina Health District," Regina: Regina Health District, 2000.
7   Susan M. Samuel, Luz Palacios-Derflingher, Marcello Tonelli, Braden Manns, Lynden Crowshoe, Sofia B. Ahmed, Min Jun, Nathalie Saad, and Brenda R. Hemmelgarn, "Association between First Nations Ethnicity and Progression to Kidney Failure by Presence and Severity of Albuminuria," *Canadian Medical Association Journal* 186, no. 2 (February 2014): E86–E94, https://doi.org/10.1503/cmaj.130776.

Indigenous people have a higher proportion of end-stage renal (kidney) disease than non-Indigenous people (33 percent of the Indigenous population with chronic kidney disease progress to dialysis, compared to 21 percent of the non-Indigenous population). The onset of chronic kidney disease is generally earlier—fifty-six years of age for the Indigenous population, versus seventy years of age for the non-Indigenous population. Since dialysis occurs at hospitals and clinics in urban centres, many Indigenous patients in Saskatchewan travel more than two hundred kilometres for dialysis treatment.[8]

Ottawa has recognized the disastrous effects of diabetes on the Indigenous population and is funding diabetes educators and public health nurses on reserves. The Canadian Diabetes Association has developed clinical practice guidelines for working with Indigenous patients.[9] One of them encourages health care professionals to "engage and connect broadly with the Indigenous community."[10] Even so, new patients often arrive in the specialist's office with untreated end-stage complications.

By late morning, the dialysis patients at the Regina General have passed through their treatment and are gathered in a waiting area inside the main door. The toxins from their failing kidneys have been filtered out, for now. Dressed in down jackets and baseball caps, they are waiting for the van to pick them up and take them home.

---

[8] Dorothy A. Thomas, Anne Huang, Michelle C.E. McCarron, Joanne I. Kappel, Rachel M. Holden, Karen E. Yeates, and Bonnie R. Richardson, "A Retrospective Study of Chronic Kidney Disease Burden in Saskatchewan's First Nations People," *Canadian Journal of Kidney Health and Disease* 5 (2018): 2054358118799689, https://doi.org/10.1177/2054358118799689.

[9] Stewart B. Harris, Onil Bhattacharyya, Roland Dyck, Mariam Naqshbandi, and Ellen L. Toth, "Type 2 Diabetes in Aboriginal Peoples," *Canadian Journal of Diabetes* 37, supplement 1 (2013): S191–S196, https://doi.org/10.1016/j.jcjd.2013.01.046.

[10] Lynden Crowshoe, David Dannenbaum, Michael Green, Rita Henderson, Mariam Naqshbandi, and Ellen Toth, "Type 2 Diabetes and Indigenous Peoples: Diabetes Canada Clinical Practice Guidelines Expert Committee," *Canadian Journal of Diabetes* 42 (2018): S296–S306, https://doi.org/10.1016/j.jcjd.2017.10.022.

+ + +

Many of my patients have blamed the diabetes epidemic on European colonization, and to some extent I agree with them. Diabetes is indeed subject to influences from the cultural and social environment.

During my first years back in Regina, I discovered that I knew very little about the Indigenous community around me. The high prevalence of diabetes concerned me, and I began to question whether the process of colonization had brought diabetes to these communities. I reviewed the journals of the explorers, Jesuit priests, and Hudson's Bay Company fur traders; none of them mentions diabetes. Diabetes was not on the radar in those days. The first survey of diabetes in Saskatchewan Indigenous populations, conducted by the Anti-Tuberculosis League of Saskatchewan in 1932, revealed no cases of diabetes in the 1,500 Indigenous people tested.[11] Judging from these records that only measured the presence of sugar in the urine, one could conclude that the disease did not manifest itself within the traditional diet and lifestyle of the Indigenous population here, likely due to subsistence living and high rates of malnutrition.

The traditional Indigenous diet, prior to the treaties and the settling of the land by European settlers, consisted of wild game like bison, elk, deer, and rabbit in addition to wild rice and berries. According to David Mandelbaum,[12] Indian turnips were the most important root food, extracted from the prairie with a digging stick. The energy expended to forage for food is estimated to be three to four thousand calories per day. Survival depended on successful hunting by the men in the community, and the harvesting and preparation of root vegetables and berries by the women and children. This lifestyle provided either plenty (after a

---

[11] Acccording to notes taken from the Records of the Saskatchewan Anti-Tuberculosis League fonds (F 535).
[12] Mandelbaum, *The Plains Cree*.

hunting expedition) or subsistence (between hunts). The expression of the diabetic trait, if present in those early days, was counteracted by high levels of physical activity and a low carb diet.

I knew that the eating habits of modern Indigenous people had changed drastically; yet it didn't make sense to me that so many were affected by diabetes. I decided to look at the underlying genetic profile that followed Indigenous people over thousands of years from Siberia to the tip of South America.

I accessed a technical internet search engine and put myself through a refresher course on the science of genes. Egg and sperm collide, and the resulting baby takes on inherited traits from both mother and father, some handed down from our distant past. Mother and father each donate twenty-three chromosomes for a total of forty-six in a normal baby. Each chromosome has multiple genes attached to it. For most genes, a complicated formula determines which of the mother's and father's traits will be expressed. If a Scot with red hair impregnates an Indigenous woman with black hair, the odds are that the gene for black hair will predominate and the gene for red hair will be suppressed. However, both genes are carried on the chromosome for life. When the child grows up and has their own children, red hair may appear in offspring or in later generations. This explains why seemingly random hair colour or texture can occur in a family after the identity of the ancestors has been all but forgotten.

The genes for diabetes are complicated. Over fifty genes have been associated with diabetes. Several studies have been done exploring the genetic factors in the Indigenous Canadian population. In a genetic survey of the population in Sandy Lake, Ontario, conducted at the end of the twenty-first century, four markers of diabetes were found.[13] Clearly,

---

13   Robert A. Hegele, Henian Cao, Stewart B. Harris, Anthony J.G. Hanley, and Bernard Zinman, "The Hepatic Nuclear Factor-1α G319S Is Associated with Early...

the study concluded, this population had a genetic predisposition to the development of diabetes, but that no one gene alone is responsible for the development of diabetes.[14]

There is debate over when the first people came to the Americas and over what period of time. One theory based on both genetic and linguistic studies suggests that a first wave arrived from the Asian landmass to the west—sometimes referred to as Beringia—and migrated throughout the two continents before the last ice age; a second wave arrived after the ice age and traveled as far as Mexico, mixing with the first wave; and a third wave, today's Inuit and related peoples, arrived more recently and settled in the far north. Whatever the genetic differences among these populations, science has been gathering evidence since at least 1965, which indicates that Indigenous Peoples of the Americas share common genetic traits linked to diabetes.[15] Perhaps the most remarkable finding, from 2007, suggests they all share a distinctive gene on chromosome 9.

A research team based at the University of California studied twenty-nine Indigenous groups from Alaska to South America and found that

---

...Onset Type-2 Diabetes in Canadian Oji-Cree," *Journal of Clinical Endocrinology & Metabolism* 84, no. 3 (March 1999): 1077–1082, https://doi.org/10.1210/jcem.84.3.5528. They discovered four gene markers suggestive of an association with diabetes (paraoxonase-2 gene, PPIR3, beta 3-adrenergic receptor, and S319 hepatic nuclear factor 1 alpha). In their study, the S319 allele is present in 20 percent of the diabetic Indigenous population.

14 Jeffrey C .Barrett, David G. Clayton, Patrick Concannon, Beena Akolkar, Jason D. Cooper, Henry A. Erlich, Cécile Julier, Grant Morahan, Jørn Nerup, Concepcion Nierras, Vincent Plagnol, Flemming Pociot, Helen Schuilenburg, Deborah J Smyth, Helen Stevens, John A. Todd, Neil M. Walker, Stephen S. Rich, and the Type 1 Diabetes Genetics Consortium, "Genome-Wide Association Study and Meta-Analysis Find That Over 40 Loci Affect Risk of Type 1 Diabetes," *Nature Genetics* 41, no. 6 (June 2009): 703–707, https://doi.org/10.1038/ng.381.

15 K.M. Venkat Narayan, "Diabetes Mellitus in Native Americans: The Problem and Its Implications," in *Changing Numbers, Changing Needs*, eds. Sandefur et al.

a unique allele "at autosomal microsatellite locus D9S1120 is present in all sampled North and South American populations, including the Na-Dene and Aleut-Eskimo, and in related Western Beringian groups, at an average frequency of 31.7%." The allele was not found in any of the sampled supposed Asian source populations or among other populations globally.[16]

The identification of the D9S1120 gene in all Indigenous people in North America and Beringia, combined with the high level of diabetes found in the Indigenous population, has strengthened the scientific consensus that there may be a genetic predisposition to the development of diabetes in Indigenous people.

I don't personally believe that it is racist to attach the term *genetic predisposition* to a genetic subgroup if it is supported by scientific evidence. There are two types of inherited disorders: single gene disorders or multifactorial. Common single gene disorders include cystic fibrosis (often found in people of European ancestry) and sickle-cell anemia (often found in people of African ancestry). Multifactorial inherited disorders are associated with a combination of genetic makeup and environment. Heart disease, for example, is widely associated in popular culture with a combination of heredity and lifestyle. Rheumatoid arthritis, another multifactorial inherited disorder, was historically seen as a disease of people from Europe. However, a recent study in Indigenous communities in Manitoba showed Indigenous people had twice the rate of rheumatoid arthritis compared to the general population.[17]

---

[16] K.B. Schroeder, T.G. Schurr, J.C. Long, N.A. Rosenberg, M.H. Crawford, L.A. Tarskaia, L.P. Osipova, S.I. Zhadanov, and D.G. Smith, "A Private Allele Ubiquitous in the Americas," *Biology Letters* 3, no. 2 (April 22, 2007): 218–223, https://doi.org/10.1098/rsbl.2006.0609.

[17] Carol A. Hitchon, Sazzadul Khan, Brend Elias, Lisa M. Lix, and Christine A. Peschken, "Prevalence and Incidence of Rheumatoid Arthritis in Canadian First Nations and Non-First Nations People: A Population-Based Study." *Journal of...*

The rate of amputation in Indigenous people is three times higher than in the white settler population.[18] Dr. David Kopriva, one of Regina General's cardiovascular surgeons, noticed in the course of his work starting around 2010, that the amputation rate in southern Saskatchewan is double the national rate. In 2019, he set out to look for a pattern. He assigned a medical student to compile a list of his surgical patients, remove the names, and then match the anonymized patients to postal codes. The results showed that many of his amputation cases came from the Touchwood Hills, an area with a concentration of Indigenous communities.

When he saw this, Dr. Kopriva contacted Susanne Nicolay at Wellness Wheel, and in the spring of 2020 he met with our team in a conference at the Regina General Hospital. He had concluded that most amputations were linked to the destructive effect of smoking on the flow of blood through the blood vessels (atherosclerosis), combined with poorly controlled diabetes. When the blood stops flowing, the affected limb—usually the leg—dies. At this meeting, he offered to work with us in an effort to reduce the amputation rate.

Health manager Val Desjarlais was intrigued by the opportunity to prevent complications of diabetes and invited Dr. Kopriva to the TATC health centre to meet patients at a Sunday lunch and join a discussion group for chronically ill residents of the area reserves. Chronic disease management is one of the pillars of tribal council funding and addresses diabetes and its complications, including kidney disease and amputations.

...*Clinical Rheumatology* 26, no. 5 (August 2020): 169–175, https://doi.org/10.1097/RHU.0000000000001006.

[18] Samuel Kwaku Essien, Gary Linassi, Margaret Larocque, and Audrey Zucker-Levin, "Incidence and Trends of Limb Amputation in First Nations and General Population in Saskatchewan, 2006–2019," *PLoS ONE* 16, no. 7 (July 12, 2021): e0254543, https://doi.org/10.1371/journal.pone.0254543.

On a Sunday morning a few months later, David and I drove north. We passed through the Qu'Appelle Valley, its tree-covered slopes awash in fog, with the red and yellow colours of fall peeping through. At the entrance to the reserve we encountered a checkpoint, set up to protect residents from casual visits during the COVID-19 pandemic.

We drove to the Touchwood Agency Tribal Council building and found a parking space at the front. As we got out of the car, a man and a woman joked with us about us not bringing COVID from the city before shaking our hands. Our COVID-19 case rate in the city had fallen to almost zero, for now, and we laughed, though somewhat nervously. The fear of city dwellers and of white people entering the safety of their lockdown was real to the people living on reserve.

It was a potluck lunch, and we had brought a fruit plate. The big boardroom featured comfy old office chairs arranged around a large central table. We put our fruit on a side table underneath public health posters promoting suicide prevention, condom use, and healthy eating. Around the table were an older couple, a single senior man, a young man with a cane sitting with his sister, and an elderly blind woman and her sister. David and I sat to the side in plastic chairs, the only chairs left in the conference room. I looked around the room for Brian, our patient from Regina who had lost his toes to amputation at the General. He was not in the room.

Val chaired the meeting. After a prayer in the Cree language blessing the land and the food, she graciously introduced us: "We are so glad that our doctors have driven from Regina to meet with us." She gave us the floor, and David talked about his research project and his wish to reduce the frequency of amputations.

I spoke about the patients from their community that I had met in the hospital, and the pleasure I always felt when I met them on reserve. I mentioned Wellness Wheel, our multidisciplinary approach, and our efforts to improve health in the community. I said that sometimes we as physicians don't know when our patients from the reserve are in hospital and said there was a need for a shared database to help track cases from the tribal council territories.

Val reclaimed the chair at this point and pointedly spoke about visiting doctors not knowing their place. I felt uncomfortable, and it appears that others at the table also felt discomfort. They looked away from her as she spoke or wiggled on their chairs. There was silence.

Then we ate: cheese, deli meats, bannock, perogies (an influence from some of the nearby settlers), and our fruit plate. Afterward, people shared more stories about their experiences in Regina and Saskatoon and their treatment in hospital—waiting in line, not being heard, complaints dismissed. It was heartfelt and upsetting, and sometimes surprising. One man told us that drowning rabbits was a cure for heart disease. David and I did not know how to respond to that revelation.

Several participants had concerns about the use of metformin, a drug that is widely prescribed to treat type 2 diabetes. One lady said that her local doctor told her to use metformin because "it was a medicine for Indians." She asked me if metformin was safe.

I tried to respond clearly to what was a complex question. There are two types of diabetes. Type 1 is sometimes called juvenile diabetes, because the person is often diagnosed in childhood and will depend on insulin for life. It results from autoimmune destruction of beta cells—the cells that produce insulin—in the pancreas. Type 1 represents approximately 10 percent of all cases of diabetes, and it is rarely inherited or linked to genetic makeup. Type 2 diabetes, representing 90 percent of cases, is associated with both inheritance and environment. As physicians, we treat type 2 diabetes with pills. If the pills stop working, we need to put our patients on insulin to control their diabetes. The presence of two types of diabetes in our human population can be confusing because both can use insulin to control their blood sugars.

Metformin is an old drug that is considered the mainstay of the treatment of non-insulin-dependent diabetes. It was originally discovered as an herb called *Galega officinalis*, also called French lilac or goat's rue, a perennial plant that grows in temperate climates. By 1923, the precise structure of the active ingredient that produced the lowering of blood glucose was shown to be the plant's galegine or isoamylene guanidine.[19] By 1977, the drug was being produced and marketed by pharmaceutical companies for the treatment of type 2 diabetes. In 1995, the seminal UK Prospective Diabetes Study demonstrated that metformin reduced the risk of heart attacks.[20] The study followed 3,800 diabetic patients over ten years. There were fewer deaths among the diabetic patients taking metformin. This study resulted in medical panels recommending metformin as the first treatment for all diabetics. As an added advantage, metformin is inexpensive, since it is generic and is not under patent protection from a drug company. It is also a safe drug. Metformin acts to control the release of glucose from the liver and does not produce low blood sugars, whereas the use of insulin for diabetes can result in dangerously low blood sugars.

"I'm not sure what your doctor meant when he said 'metformin is for Indians,'" I said. "He may have been referring to your people's propensity to develop diabetes." I tried to reassure her that it might not be her fault that she was diabetic, given that the genes for diabetes are inherited.

She listened politely, but she seemed troubled. At the time, I was not aware of the rejection of genetic predisposition for health conditions among Indigenous people. On reflection, I realize that my words may have been interpreted as condescending, paternalistic, and judgmental.

---

19 Clifford J. Bailey, "Metformin: Historical Overview," *Diabetologia* 60, no. 9 (September 2017): 1566–1576, https://doi.org/10.1007/s00125-017-4318-z.
20 U.K. Prospective Diabetes Study Group, "U.K. Prospective Diabetes Study 16: Overview of 6 Years' Therapy of Type II Diabetes: A Progressive Disease," *Diabetes* 44, no. 11 (November 1, 1995): 1249–1258, https://doi.org/10.2337/diab.44.11.1249.

I had been trying so hard to be culturally sensitive, using two-eyed seeing to inform my interactions. Despite my attempts at reconciliation, there was much more I needed to learn to achieve true reconciliation.

There was silence, and then Val spoke up.

"You can't put candy in front of our people. It's because they don't eat right. There is no such thing as a diabetic gene. We need to get the balance in our community and put our faith in the Creator."

I believed I was an expert in this area, but I had been effectively muzzled by the group leader. She was establishing control with a bias that refused to accept my view of the scientific evidence. In her view, spiritual balance must precede physical balance. Val was affirming the importance of spirituality. I acquiesced to her conviction that if the ways of the Creator had been followed, then these modern illnesses would not necessarily have happened. Again, the settlers had disrupted Indigenous philosophy and practices that promoted harmony and healing.

Focus groups in Indigenous communities describe the following common themes: Diabetes is the consequence of the loss of traditional ways, not living a "right life," or breaking a spirit-imposed taboo. Diabetes is a "white man's sickness" and results from disruption of the tribal way of life and contamination of the environment and food supply by white people. Some believe that diabetes is contagious and can infect weak people.[21]

The science linked to genetic testing has come into disrepute partly because of the confusion caused by online testing services such as MyHeritage.com or Ancestry.com.[22] Easy genetic testing services have

---

21   Kelly Acton, "Alternative and Complementary Approaches to Diabetes: Where Is the Evidence for the Native American Population," presentation given at the American Diabetes Association's 66th Annual Meeting and Scientific Sessions in Washington, DC, 2006.
22   For further reading in this area, see Charles Seife, "23andMe Is Terrifying, but Not for the Reasons the FDA Thinks: The Genetic-Testing Company's Real Goal Is to...

affected the authenticity of blood quotient determination for Indigenous Peoples. There have been a flood of users trying to prove tribal claims or gain treaty status. So, genetics is important in some cases, but there is an alternative view of the science of genetic testing. There is a traditional view that susceptibility to disease is the work of the Creator, and not of our genes. Indigenous anthropologist Kim TallBear told the *New Scientist* in 2014, "There are also traditional people who don't want to have a molecular narrative of history shoved down their throats. They would prefer to privilege the tribal creation stories that root us in the landscapes we come from."[23]

David and I sat back and accepted our beating. We left shortly after, and we discussed diabetes in the car on the way home. Approximately 14 percent of Indigenous people have diabetes, compared with only 4 percent of non-Indigenous Canadians. The facts are clear that undiagnosed and poorly treated diabetes is a major contributor to poor health and early death. The issue for us was how to engage the patients in self-care to prevent the complications. David and I concluded that it was going to be difficult to reduce the rate of amputation in this community.

...Hoard Your Personal Data," *Scientific American*, November 27, 2013, https://www.scientificamerican.com/article/23andme-is-terrifying-but-not-for-the-reasons-the-fda-thinks/.

23   Linda Geddes, "'There Is No DNA Test to Prove You're Native American,'" *New Scientist*, February 5, 2014, https://www.newscientist.com/article/mg22129554-400-there-is-no-dna-test-to-prove-youre-native-american/#ixzz75bnfcEBi.

ANXIETY

The health clinic is closed today. The other services on reserve are closed as well: schools, band office, store, and gas station. It is a day of mourning. This day becomes another cultural learning moment for me and Stu.

We have enjoyed a sunny two-hour drive from Regina. Stu gets a phone call from the clinic health director. We are a few minutes from our destination. We learn that there has been a death in the community, and everyone who works at the clinic is related to the deceased in some way. When someone dies, the relatives who live on reserve attend a wake. Appointments with patients are cancelled. The wake will continue until nightfall—a solemn and ceremonial event, and a social occasion at the same time. The deceased was not one of our patients and is unknown to us. Stu and I discuss the situation: the patients whom we would have seen at the clinic that day will have to wait until our next visit. Despite our connection to the health of the community, we recognize that we are not part of the community. We feel uncomfortable attending the wake, since we do not know the deceased. We turn the car around and go back to the city.

In my work as a doctor, I deal with death almost every day. Physicians are trained to do everything to prolong life, but eventually every patient dies. There are innumerable patterns in death—sudden death from a heart attack, self-inflicted death, death from preventable or accidental trauma, death from metastatic cancer, death from medical error, prolonged death, agonizing death, peaceful death in old age. Each patient is on their own path, physically and mentally. With each case that I witness, I am affected by my own form of grieving. It can be silent resignation to the eventual presence of the grim reaper, or sadness at the loss, or spiritual thoughts about an afterlife. At other times I have been affected by the unfortunate end of life from metastatic cancer in a young person, or trauma, or suicide, or murder. As a physician, I remember the deceased patients I have known—their spirits stay with me. Publicly I carefully monitor my reaction, but internally I suffer spiritually from loss of life.

Carol, an administrator at one of the band offices in the Touchwood Hills, has told me about her Indigenous name. In a Sweat Ceremony, she was given her name, which means something approximating "the one that guards the cemetery." She cannot translate it exactly—there is no English word to describe her role. She sees spirits from the cemetery. They come to visit her every night. They come into her bedroom and dance around her. She tells me that the medication that I have given her to aid with sleep has helped her avoid these interruptions. When she takes the medication, her nocturnal visions disappear. I recognize that I have relieved her burden of guarding the cemetery in the community, but I confess to her that I am troubled with the imposition of non-Indigenous, pharmaceutical sleep medication on her traditional role. We spend some time discussing the pros and cons of the integration of Western medicine in Indigenous life. We finally decided that she will take the medication intermittently. Maintaining my emotional distance to adhere to professionalism, I do not tell her how I feel about cemeteries or how I feel after I experience a patient's death.

Indigenous people see death frequently from an early age. Federal briefing documents from 2019 reveal that life expectancy for Indigenous in Canada is fifteen years shorter than for other Canadians.[1] Most of my patients talk to me about these losses. For some, the number of events is so high that I wonder how they withstand the barrage of tragedy. The uncle who died from kidney failure after years of uncontrolled diabetes. The father who died of a heart attack precipitated by untreated hypertension. The loss of an unborn child after an absence of prenatal care. The death of a husband from gunfire during an elk hunt in the Touchwood Hills. The fatal shooting of a loved one outside a bar in any one of a dozen cities. The suicide of a teenager who believes there is no hope. The overdoses from fentanyl.

My patients may talk about the death of this or that relative, but they almost never talk about the looming presence of death in general with me. Virtually every Indigenous family carries scars from Canada's residential school system. There are still many people alive who passed through the system and survived it, and there are many others, younger people, who have suffered crippling trauma related to the experiences of their parents or grandparents. This trauma continues to cause severe anxiety, which in turn interferes with rational decision-making. The medical profession has created a narrative that results in the medicalization of trauma. When they appear in the ER, the medical model makes the resilient community members into victims of institutional racism disregarding the personal background of family members who have died from inadequate prenatal care, from TB, Hep C, HIV, or syphilis epidemics, and from lack of access to care.

---

1   Michael Tjepkema, Tracey Bushnik, and Evelyne Bougie, "Life Expectancy of First Nations, Métis and Inuit Household Populations in Canada," Statistics Canada Health Reports, December 18, 2019, https://www.doi.org/10.25318/82-003-x201901200001-eng.

Imagine a child of residential school Survivors growing up in North Central Regina. One notorious effect of the city schools, along with the loss of language and culture, is the economic reality of survival. Their parents, with little opportunity for education on reserve, have moved into the city and work as garbage collectors, waiters, or hotel cleaners. They take classes at night to further their education. Sometimes, their kôhkom, or grandmother, lives with them to maintain stability. Even so, regardless of personalities, family support, or strength of character, it is likely that the wage earner's employment is insecure and their food supply is uncertain. The socio-economic reality is that they live in a rented house in a precarious, often dangerous part of the city. The child may see shootings and suicides up and down the block, people acting out their mental health struggles, police officers and strangers coming to the door.

The typical human response in a high-stress situation is to make a choice between fight or flight. As one American pediatrician expressed: "If you're in a forest and see a bear, a very efficient fight-or-flight system instantly floods your body with adrenaline and cortisol and shuts off the thinking portion of your brain that would stop to consider other options. This is very helpful if you're in a forest and you need to run from a bear."[2] However, when the bear comes into the house every day, the child is trained into a permanent state of fight-or-flight.

Here's a slightly more technical explanation for anxiety. Humans have evolved to survive using skills that reside in many parts of the brain. These skills include vision and hearing, perceptual skills to measure the physical and emotional environment, physical control over muscle functions, and problem-solving, all of which allows a person to access what they need to survive.

---

2   Nadine Burke Harris quoted in "Back to School," *This American Life* episode 474, September 14, 2012, produced by Ben Calhoun, Sarah Koenig, and Ira Glass, Public Radio International, https://www.thisamericanlife.org/474/transcript.

The occipital lobe at the back of the brain is often called the eyes in the back of the head because it processes visual stimuli from the environment. The frontal lobe controls planning and problem-solving. The limbic system, seated deep in the inner part of the brain, processes emotions and sends signals to other parts of the brain to influence behaviour.

The limbic system controls our responses to environmental stimuli such as physical threats (an armed man confronting you in a back alley), social disruption (watching your parent being beaten in a case of domestic violence), and emotional abuse (derogatory comments from a parent to their teenage offspring). This system is the seat of emotions like fear, anxiety, reward, and attraction.[3] It controls the flight, flight, or freeze hormones in the body and brain. If the stimulus is short term, the resulting changes in the brain function recover. When the stimulus is persistent and severe, there can be long-lasting changes to the brain that result in hypersensitivity of the limbic system and a tendency towards chronic anxiety.

Brain scans in people with anxiety show changes in the brain. The amygdala, part of the limbic system of the brain, is activated. Greater activity in the amygdala correlates with increased cortisol and a higher risk for heart disease and stroke.[4] Stimulation of this part of the brain can also shut down normal bodily functions, like the sleep cycle, appetite, and motivation to exercise. It also results in the decision to self-medicate to relieve the symptoms.

---

[3] Katie Sokolowski and Joshua G. Corbin, "Wired for Behaviors: From Development to Function of Innate Limbic System Circuitry," *Frontiers in Molecular Neuroscience* 5, no. 55 (April 26, 2012), https://doi.org/10.3389/fnmol.2012.00055.

[4] Yuko Hakamata, Shotaro Komi, Yoshiya Moriguchi, Shuhei Izawa, Yuki Motomura, Eisuke Sato, Shinya Mizukami, Yoshiharu Kim, Takashi Hanakawa, Yusuke Inoue, and Hirokuni Tagaya, "Amygdala-Centred Functional Connectivity Affects Daily Cortisol Concentrations: A Putative Link with Anxiety," *Scientific Reports* 7, no. 8313 (August 16, 2017), https://doi.org/10.1038/s41598-017-08918-7.

The *Diagnostic and Statistical Manual of Mental Disorders* defines the effects of trauma in medical terms as post-traumatic stress disorder (PTSD).[5] People with PTSD exhibit physical symptoms that get reactivated or triggered when the trauma wound is stimulated by an internal or external cue. These physical symptoms include a racing heart, increased breathing rate, stomach pain, dizziness, headache, and chest pain. Anxiety is linked to PTSD, activating similar areas of the brain.[6] It is often difficult for a physician to tease out the physical symptoms from the psychological trigger, since it is difficult for the patient to explain the link between trauma and the physical complaints. Often, these patients end up receiving a lot of investigations and medical interventions.

Since the 1980s, researchers have been looking at the relationship of adult mental health disorders and adverse childhood experiences (ACE) in three major categories: abuse, neglect, and household dysfunction. Children with high levels of exposure to adversity are more than four times as likely to develop a mental health disorder by the time they reach adulthood than children who have not experienced adversity.[7] Nearly eight hundred scientific articles have been written about ACEs over the last twenty years.[8]

---

[5] Matthew J. Friedman, Patricia A. Resick, Richard A. Bryant, James Strain, Mardi Horowitz, and David Spiegel, "Classification of Trauma and Stressor-Related Disorders in DSM-5," *Depression and Anxiety* 28, no. 9 (September 2011): 737–749, https://doi.org/10.1002/da.20845.

[6] David J. Nutt and Andrea L. Malizia, "Structural and Functional Brain Changes in Posttraumatic Stress Disorder," *The Journal of Clinical Psychiatry* 65, suppl. 1 (2004): 11–7, https://pubmed.ncbi.nlm.nih.gov/14728092/.

[7] Katie A. McLaughlin, Jennifer Greif Green, Michael J. Gruber, Nancy A. Sampson, Alan M. Zaslavsky, and Ronald C. Kessler," Childhood Adversities and First Onset of Psychiatric Disorders in a National Sample of Adolescents," *Archives of General Psychiatry* 69, no. 11 (November 1, 2012): 1151–1160, https://doi.org/10.1001/archgenpsychiatry.2011.2277.

[8] Shannon Struck, Ashley Stewart-Tufescu, Aleiia J.N. Asmundson, Gordon G.J. Asmundson, and Tracie O. Afifi, "Adverse Childhood Experiences (ACEs)...

Cultural assimilation policies, typified by American Civil War veteran Richard H. Pratt's phrase "Kill the Indian in him, and save the man,"[9] had disastrous effects on the limbic system. Many Indigenous children who were taken from their traditional homes and sent to residential schools experienced mistreatment, overwork, and denial of basic needs such as food, and they were taught that Indian ways were shameful. Some were subjected to, or witnessed, brutal physical, sexual, verbal, and psychological abuse.[10] Students left these schools disassociated from their traditional culture with a lack of identity and an inability to form meaningful interpersonal relationships. The trauma resulted in chronic anxiety, substance abuse, conflicts with authority, and the inability to integrate into either their traditional culture or the dominant settler community. The children of school Survivors witnessed this self-destructive behaviour, feeding a vicious cycle of intergenerational neglect, abuse, aggression, self-harm, and trauma.[11]

Love and support were the mainstay of my childhood. My teenage years were relatively carefree. I didn't understand debilitating anxiety

---

...Research: A Bibliometric Analysis of Publication Trends over the First 20 Years," *Child Abuse & Neglect* 112, article 104895 (February 2021), https://doi.org/10.1016/j.chiabu.2020.104895. One of the authors in this study, Gordon Asmundson, is local to Saskatchewan, in the Department of Psychology and Anxiety at the University of Regina.

9   R.H. Pratt, "The Advantages of Mingling Indians with Whites," in Isabel C. Barrows, ed., *Proceedings of the National Conference of Charities and Correction at the 19th Annual Session Held in Denver, Col., June 23–29, 1892* (Boston, 1892), 45–59, https://carlisleindian.dickinson.edu/sites/default/files/docs-resources/CIS-Resources_1892-PrattSpeech.pdf

10   William Aguiar and Regine Halseth, "Aboriginal Peoples and Historic Trauma: The Processes of Intergenerational Transmission," National Collaborating Centre for Aboriginal Health, 2015, https://www.ccnsa-nccah.ca/docs/context/RPT-HistoricTrauma-IntergenTransmission-Aguiar-Halseth-EN.pdf.

11   Amrita Roy, "Intergenerational Trauma and Aboriginal Women: Implications for Mental Health During Pregnancy," *First Peoples Child & Family Review* 9, no. 1 (October 1, 2014), 7–21, https://doi.org/10.7202/1071790ar.

until quite recently—and my discovery arose from a situation where there was no obvious cause for anxiety because there was no obvious threat.

My father died on October 31, 2018, seven years after I returned to Regina. His death was expected. For two years prior to his death, I sat with him each day in his room at a very comfortable long-term care home in one of the new suburbs of Regina. In winter, we watched curling together on his television. He had a prairie pride in his curling experience and knew every strategy and move on the ice. *Our team blanked the end. We got the hammer. That rock curled over the hog line. Are they going to freeze or raise? Wow, right on the button.* We cheered together when one team or another hit a double or triple out of the house. We lived in the present moment. When the game was over and the nursing staff came into his room and put him to bed, he would look at me and say, "I wonder if tonight is going to be the night." And he would look into my eyes knowingly and deep, with resignation. He was a hundred years old. He was prepared for death and let me know that death was imminent.

He died in his sleep. My brother called me at 4:00 a.m. to let me know that he had heard from the care home. There were arrangements to be made, preparing the body for cremation, collecting the personal items cleaned out from his now-empty room. My father, ever the economist, had timed his death for the last day of the month; we did not have to pay for any unused days. We got busy with the details. Four days after his death, I began to experience anxiety.

It was anxiety as I had never experienced it before. Prior to this, I had defined anxiety as the feeling you have when traffic is bad on the way to the airport and you worry about missing your plane. Butterflies in your stomach, the shutdown of pleasant thoughts, a total focus on each red light. Then you get to the airport and the lines are short. You pass through security, arriving at the gate with twenty minutes to spare. The anxiety subsides, and life goes on.

I didn't shed tears after my father's death. I had expected it and he was ready for it, so there was only a slight feeling of loss, or so I thought. He had lived a long and successful life that I had celebrated with my family, friends, and community. In a sense, freedom was in front of me. I had relinquished my commitments in the US to concentrate on writing this book. I was free of parental responsibility. I looked forward to having more time for other pursuits now that my visits with my father had ended. I told my friends I was planning to attend a writing retreat.

The anxiety started with a low-level rumbling stomach ache in the morning. I ate breakfast and planned my day. I sat down in front of my computer. By noon, the rumbling had intensified. I found it difficult to concentrate, so I dropped my goal-oriented writing and switched to arts and crafts and talking to friends on the phone. By late afternoon my anxiety was raging to the point that I couldn't do anything: I couldn't concentrate on cooking supper for myself, and when I called another friend, my speech was rapid and disconnected. I tried to calm down with yoga (couldn't breathe normally). I tried to calm down with an outdoor walk (got lost in my own neighbourhood). I tried an alcoholic drink (which increased the anxiety). I tried television (every show was boring). I tried a book (couldn't focus). Eventually, I took a sleeping pill and dozed off without undressing.

The pattern repeated the next day. My anxiety increased through the day to the point where I couldn't stand being in my own skin. It happened again the next day, and the next. After a couple of weeks, I had talked with all my family and friends about my father's death and sent out emails and thank-you notes. But the anxiety continued. It was fight or flight—but flight from what?

I signed up for the HBO network and binge-watched drama series until I fell asleep on the couch. Some days I was overwhelmed and couldn't even manage TV. I finally arranged to meet with my friend Mary Lou, a spiritual therapist. I told her about the anxiety that was paralyzing me. She calmly looked at me and said, "You're grieving the loss of your father. Live with it, feel it, experience it. It will pass as your soul adjusts to the loss."

Naming the problem helped me to turn the corner. I began to feel better. After another month, I was still experiencing low-level anxiety every morning, but it didn't escalate. I began to get some things accomplished. I could do yoga, take a walk, read a book. I attended the writing retreat and returned to work at the Regina General Hospital. By the third month, my anxiety was barely noticeable. Then, suddenly, it was gone. I was my normal self again.

My patients sometimes talk to me about their anxiety. I'm not a psychotherapist, but especially since I had my own experience of losing my way, I see the link between crippling anxiety and an inability to make decisions. All of my colleagues who work with anxious patients, Indigenous or non-Indigenous, see a pattern of skipped appointments and a failure to take medications or to practise basic self-care.

I can imagine a patient describing their experience of anxiety: "I try to make sense of it. I try to understand why it comes up again and again, but I can't grab onto it. It's like a cloud swirling around inside. It's like an energy coming up from the floor and making my heart run faster. If one part of me wants to get dressed to go out; the other part is telling me to sit still and wait. Other doctors have told me to try to figure out where it started. Like they think my life is a straight line with all the dots connected. I don't know why I have to be like this."

But while my Indigenous patients may talk about their struggle with anxiety, they almost never talk about their family experience with residential schools. It seems that for the most part they have never felt safe in talking about it, or they have not found the vocabulary or given themselves permission. Or maybe it is the settler-Indigenous relationship that is unstated but present in every interaction? I have learned over time to assume that residential school trauma is there, waiting in the background. In 2019, a year after my father's death, as I sat in a lecture hall at the University of Regina, I listened to Connie Walker, the keynote speaker at the thirty-eighth annual Minifie Lecture, say "remember the context." Her statement resonates with me almost every day.

When the Canadian news media reported the discovery of unmarked children's graves in various parts of Western Canada in the summer of 2021, it raised public awareness about the residential schools and the misery they had caused. For over 160 years, there were more than 140 residential schools that operated in Canada, until the last closed in 1996, practising a systematic neglect that led to the deaths of unknown thousands of children.[12] Twenty schools in Saskatchewan were operated by the Roman Catholic Church, the Anglicans, the United Church, and the Presbyterians. The United Church of Canada apologized in 1986; the Anglican Church of Canada in 1993; and the Presbyterian Church of Canada in 1994.[13] Their apology goes like this:

> I accept and I confess before God and you, our failures in the residential schools. We failed you. We failed ourselves. We failed God. I am sorry, more than I can say, that we were part of a system which took you and your children from home and family. I am sorry, more than I can say, that we tried to remake you in our image, taking from you your language and the signs of your identity. I am sorry, more than I

---

12 On July 1, 2021, CBC News reported that there was an estimate of six thousand dead, but this number was expected to rise. Ka'nhehsí:io Deer, "Why It's Difficult to Put a Number on How Many Children Died at Residential Schools," CBC News, September 29, 2021, https://www.cbc.ca/news/indigenous/residential-school-children-deaths-numbers-1.6182456.

13 Links to apologies offered by the Anglican, Presbyterian, and United Churches and the Government of Canada can be found online at https://projectofheart.ca/apologies/. Other institutions that have offered apologies include the Government of Alberta (2015), the Government of Ontario (2016), and the Royal Canadian Mounted Police (2019).

can say, that in our schools so many were abused physically, sexually, culturally and emotionally.

The Canadian Conference of Catholic Bishops apologized twenty-seven years later,[14] and the global head of the Catholic Church, Pope Francis, apologized in Rome to a delegation of Indigenous people from Turtle Island in April 2022.

In the summer of the discovery of the unmarked graves, my phone was ringing off the hook. American friends who read the *New York Times*[15] and other local news sources called me to express concern about news that unmarked graves had been found at residential schools in Canada. The graves were decades old and were identified through the use of radar technology. It was an international embarrassment for a Trudeau Liberal government that had endorsed the findings of the Truth and Reconciliation Commission in 2016. I was surprised that my American friends were paying attention, but I quickly realized that this news had been amplified around the world by the mainstream press and social media.

Weeks after the news from Kamloops, the discovery of more than seven hundred unmarked graves at the site of the Marieval Indian Residential School on the Cowessess First Nation in Saskatchewan triggered a visceral reaction in my gut. I have visited this place. It is just over an hour's drive east of Regina. The number is horrific, and yet very few people knew. The parents of those children knew. The Truth and Reconciliation Commission knew and asked for funding to investigate. The previous federal government led by Conservative Stephen Harper denied them funding.

---

14 Reuters, "Catholic Bishops in Canada Apologize for Indigenous Residential Schools," NBC News, September 25, 2021, https://www.nbcnews.com/news/world/catholic-bishops-canada-apologize-indigenous-residential-schools-n1280082.
15 Ian Austen, "How Thousands of Indigenous Children Vanished in Canada," *The New York Times*, March 28, 2022, https://www.nytimes.com/2021/06/07/world/canada/mass-graves-residential-schools.html.

The work accomplished with ground-penetrating radar technology at the school sites validates the assertions that Indigenous people have discussed for decades. In 2018, I sat down with Doug Stewart after the publication of his book about the Regina Indian Industrial School.[16] The school closed in 1910 after about twenty years in operation and was forgotten by the general public until 2012, when a campaign was initiated to restore and preserve the school cemetery just west of Regina. As a result of this campaign, the site received provincial and municipal heritage status. There are only two burials, however, with a marker, and that marker commemorates the children of a school principal. There are at least forty more unmarked graves containing the bodies of Indigenous students. Some graves likely contain more than one body.

"We've spent a lot of time justifying these deaths," Doug said to me. "Government policy in the late 1800s was to promote integration into white settler society. I searched through the school records in the Saskatchewan archives, but there isn't much to document the deaths. There were very few medical services available between 1891 and 1910. For heaven's sake, we didn't even have a hospital in Regina until 1905, and it was a cottage hospital. Infectious diseases bred and spread like wildfire in those cramped residential dormitories. We don't need to imagine that the children died from beatings, even if corporal punishment was the norm. They died from poverty."

If the children had been white, I believe the truth would have surfaced many years earlier. For example, authorities reacted immediately to the "Butterbox Babies" scandal in the 1940s. The operation of a home for unwed mothers in Atlantic Canada resulted in the deaths of between four hundred and six hundred infants. The operators collected fees to care for ostracized pregnant girls. If the newborn infants

---

16 Douglas Stewart, *The Regina Indian Industrial School (1891–1910): Historical Overview and Chronological Narrative* (Regina: Benchmark Press, 2017).

were not adopted after birth, they were neglected and starved. When they died, they were placed in pine butter crates and buried. The trial of a midwife and a Seventh Day Adventist pastor led to the closure of the home in 1946 along with widespread publicity and expressions of horror.

Over most of Canada's history, some Indigenous children watched their brothers and sisters die in the residential schools. Now that the conditions in the schools are common knowledge, my American friends ask again and again: How did so many die? Were they beaten to death? Did they die from communicable diseases like TB, measles, and influenza? We don't know the answer. The link between poverty and reduced life expectancy provides some explanation. Reports from medical surveys in the 1890 to 1910 period show that Indigenous people were more vulnerable to disease compared to the white settler population. Epidemics of typhoid, influenza, and measles killed hundreds of children, especially those at residential schools. Malnutrition is associated with an accelerated death rate in response to measles. Tuberculosis spread quickly in the cramped multigenerational conditions on reserves, with children carrying the tuberculin bacillus to the residential schools where they infected others.

Vincent Steinhauer, past president of University nuhelot'įne thaiyots'į nistameyimâkanak Blue Quills, an Alberta-based Indigenous college, has the following perspective from his position of Indigenous governance:

> Europeans broke the first law of "love" when they abducted Indigenous children into residential schools and caused loss of hope across generations. Indigenous people were given many spiritual laws to guide their relationships with all life. A child-rearing law is *opikinawasowin* (Cree word for nurturing our children well). Children are sacred gifts from the creator, and ceremonies were embedded at each phase of their life—by protocol they were welcomed into this

world, embraced by community as spiritual beings, and celebrated in ceremonies with each stage of development. So much has been lost in practice but remains in genetic memory. Elder wisdom is still available for happy, healthy and sustainable futures.[17]

In the Judeo-Christian bible, suffering originates with Adam and Eve's ejection from the Garden of Eden. Through the interpretation of this creation story, the Doctrine of Discovery was used to justify rejecting Indigenous wisdom. The Indigenous view holds that creation was a gift and privilege that humans needed to respect and nurture.[18]

North American white society, like many other societies around the world, has seen a high incidence of post-traumatic stress disorder through the wars of the past 150 years. However, the problem was rarely named, or at least it was not taken seriously. It was a sign of moral weakness for a returning soldier to experience chronic after-effects from violence. Not until the current century and the appearance of numerous articles, documentaries, and popular books such as Bessel van der Kolk's *The Body Keeps the Score*[19] did an understanding of traumatic stress become an aspect of everyday reality and consciousness.

The popular acceptance of the reality of PTSD has helped create a political space where Canadian governments are able to achieve

---

17 Gregory A. Cajete, "Children, Myth and Storytelling: An Indigenous Perspective," *Global Studies of Childhood* 7, no. 2 (June 2017), 113–130, https://doi.org/10.1177/2043610617703832. Vincent Steinhauer died at age fifty-four from a sudden heart attack on Febuary 25, 2019. Julia Lipscombe and Ariel Fournier, "Community Mourns Beloved Cree Educator, Leader and 'Truth Teller,'" CBC News, March 1, 2019, https://www.cbc.ca/news/canada/edmonton/cree-educator-vincent-steinhauer-dies-1.5039722.
18 Personal conversation in June through August of 2022 with Blair Stonechild, author of *Loss of Indigenous Eden and the Fall of Spirituality* (Regina: University of Regina Press, 2020).
19 Bessel Van der Kolk, *The Body Keeps the Score: Brain, Mind, and Body in the Healing of Trauma* (New York: Penguin Books, 2015).

financial settlements with residential school Survivors and their families. Ottawa's Indian Residential Schools Settlement Agreement was implemented in 2007, following decades of pressure from Indigenous organizations. An official report issued in 2021 stated that up until that year the Independent Assessment Process had ordered 27,846 awards at a total value of $3.233 billion.[20] This was in addition to an estimated $1.622 billion paid out to almost eighty thousand claimants under an earlier Common Experience Payment program.[21] Programs are also available for people who need emotional support, such as through the Indian Residential Schools Resolution Health Support Program. Any relative of a residential school Survivor can receive funding for professional counselling, emotional support, and reimbursement for transportation.

One day recently, I had the opportunity to see the legal document from the Indian Residential Schools Settlement. One of my patients showed me a letter from his TRC lawyer. The letter stated, in bold print, that he was entitled to receive $50,000. My patient asked me how he could leverage this letter to obtain immediate cash for living expenses, essentially asking me for a loan. He was earnest and truthful. I believed in him, knowing that he would pay me back when the funds arrived. I knew that he was just trying to survive until the money came in and that he was not aware that he was being manipulative. In response, I had to tell him that I was his doctor, and it was not appropriate for me to also be his bank.

Mainstream society has a history of resisting funding for empowerment programs to strengthen Indigenous communities. Given the

---

[20] Independent Assessment Process Oversight Committee, *Independent Assessment Process Final Report*, 2021, http://www.iap-pei.ca/media/information/publication/pdf/FinalReport/IAP-FR-2021-03-11-eng.pdf.

[21] "Statistics on the Implementation of the Indian Residential Schools Settlement Agreement," Government of Canada, https://www.rcaanc-cirnac.gc.ca/eng/1315320539682/1571590489978.

direct costs of these programs and the social costs generated by the residential schools over time, it would have been wiser for the treaty makers and federal governments instead to support and strengthen Indigenous communities by offering housing, health care, and access to areas of traditional land use. It would have saved money in the long run to have invested resources into land claims, housing, education, and health care. That could have happened in 1876 when Chiefs Poundmaker, Mistawasis, and Ahtahkakoop requested it. It could have happened in 1945 if Mackenzie King had not cut the budget of Indian Affairs. It could have happened in 1966 when the Hawthorn Report proposed that all forced assimilation programs, such as the residential schools, should be abolished, and that Aboriginal peoples should be seen as "citizens plus"—with the opportunities and resources for self-determination.[22] The phrase "citizens plus" resulted in Pierre Trudeau's White Paper in 1971—a fiasco of a paper, which suggested assimilation tactics, further widening the settler-Indigenous divide. It could have happened in 1982 when Section 35 of the Constitution Act recognized Indigenous and treaty rights, including the treaty right to health.[23] Yet, health is narrowly defined and does not embody cultural wellness and a holistic approach that is implied in the Medicine Wheel. Numerous historical mistakes have been committed by misguided government policies. No wonder the 1876 Indian Act is reviled. We have a big problem on our hands.

Indigenous organizations, with support from local communities and government budgets, are working to heal the Survivors of the

---

22 H.B. Hawthorn, ed., *A Survey of the Contemporary Indians of Canada: A Report on Economic, Political, Educational Needs and Policies in Two Volumes* (Ottawa: Indian Affairs Branch, 1966, publication no. QS-0603-020-EE-A-18), https://caid.ca/HawRep1a1966.pdf.

23 "Section 35 Aboriginal and Treaty Rights," Centre for Constitutional Studies, September 9, 2021, https://www.constitutionalstudies.ca/2021/09/section-35-aboriginal-and-treaty-rights/.

residential schools and their families, through traditional healing circles and the education of Indigenous people as therapists and doctors. However, as the saying goes, the body keeps score. The effects of experiences that no one ever talked about are still emerging among my patients in the form of stomach ailments, heart ailments, cancers, and mental breakdown.

Since my return to Saskatchewan in 2011 I have cared for patients from all demographic and social backgrounds. I have worked with military veterans from settler families who suffered deeply from battle-related post-traumatic stress. I've treated immigrant patients who lost everything in civil wars in Asia and Africa, barely escaping after watching the slaughter of their relatives and neighbours. The effects from these experiences may be manageable, or they may continue to drive physical illness, psychosis, family dysfunction, and in some cases suicide. My Indigenous patients are distinct in the world of the traumatized because of their lifelong exposure to traumatizing events. This has led to profound anxiety, with the sheer number of sufferers making up entire sections of Canada's prairie cities. Their trauma has been sponsored to a large extent by Canadian governments, churches, and other established institutions. The holistic view of individual and communal health, as defined by the medicine chest clause, has been infringed upon by both provincial and federal government agencies.

FOOD ON THE RESERVE

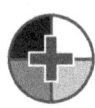

I am a prairie girl who does not mind winter. I have pleasant childhood memories of crunchy snow and sparkling air. I've always had confidence that our electrical network and natural gas furnaces will stand the test and keep me warm and cozy if I stay inside. And even without electric power or natural gas, a brief time living off the grid taught me that an axe, a woodpile, and a wood-burning stove in an insulated house are enough to survive the cold.

As Susanne and I are driving to one of the Touchwood communities on a morning in January, it's minus forty degrees. The sun is bright; there are crystals in the air. We are driving in a warm car along a paved highway, protected from the elements. I look at the wind-swept prairie, deep snow on the fields, hollows with bare stunted trees—they might provide some shelter, but not enough to survive. My mind wanders. What would it be like to live without the infrastructure that settler communities built here? What was it like when my ancestors huddled in their sod houses? What was it like before that? How did the Indigenous people cope with this cold?[1]

---

1   Part of the answer to how they survived such cold winters is that Indigenous people travelled south as far as they could, or west to such relatively "warm"...

We encounter a row of wooden framed houses along a dirt road at the entrance to our host community. Each house is different, but they all show the stamp of government issue—administered by the elected local council but built on a plan developed in Ottawa. They are wooden and square. One has new yellow paint, another is half painted. The yellow one has three wooden steps going to a white front door, which is pock-marked from the scratching of a dog's nails. Another house is painted in a colour that blends into the grey-blue sky. Its broken front windows are covered with plywood, while a side window consists of a plastic sheet. Beside a house farther along, I see a broken-down car with its engine hood open and tires flat. A rusted children's swing is set off to the side of a fourth house, its broken seat flopping in the wind at the end of a tarnished chain. There are no fences, no defined yards, no property lines. Garbage is littered around one house, some in bags, some strewn over the yard. The wind is cold and blustery. The houses look empty, but how can you tell? There is no one walking on the road. The first people we see are sitting in cars in the village, either on the street or in the parking lot at the health centre. They appear to be smoking.

As we enter the health clinic with our travelling medicine chest, I say hello to Roxane Wagner. She has been the Aboriginal Diabetes Initiative worker in this community since 2015, the year before we started Wellness Wheel. She is a bright-eyed forty-year-old non-Indigenous woman with an engaging spirit. She now lives on a farm down the road where she grew up. Prior to this, she had extensive professional experience grappling with nutrition and food security issues, both internationally and in Toronto's inner city. She loves her work, and I am learning that she is sensitive to the Indigenous narrative style

---

...places as the Cypress Hills, following the bison, where they wintered in tipis with buffalo skin blankets.

and gets along well with the local community. She invites me to attend a diabetes teaching group session this morning. Since there are no patients yet in the clinic and my list is empty for the moment, I agree to observe the class—with the proviso that I will let myself out as soon as a patient arrives.

We find ten women around the table in the conference room, ranging in age from twenty to seventy years. All have diabetes, and they are here to learn about how to manage their conditions. Roxane leads the group with a gentle style and elicits their participation. She asks: What is a carbohydrate? A voice from around the table says potatoes. Another one says bannock. Roxane says: What about fruit? I smile because it is a trick question. Most people don't recognize fruit as a carbohydrate—it is a "free" food in the Weight Watchers list, but it contains sugars that can spike the blood sugars. There is no judgment in the room, but I sense a disconnect among the participants. Knowledge is one thing, implementation is another, especially when the one store in the community sells only snack foods. And everyone likes fruit.

There is no café on the reserve. I have forgotten my packed lunch, and at noon I drive the two city blocks to the corner store to see what I can find. The store sells gas, cigarettes, chips, soda pop, and candy. Its front door has two padlocks, but today the door swings open easily to an area of shelves and low lighting. Near the cash register, a hot dog roller has a few hot dogs slowly rotating on its burner next to a stack of buns and a mustard squeeze bottle. Behind me is a shelf of chips, all varieties, and in the corner, a cooler with Coke, Pepsi, 7-Up, Gatorade, and water in bottles. I am actually looking forward to a hot dog—I rarely eat them, so they are always a treat. I buy one, slather it with mustard, and pick up a bottle of water as well. I go back to the clinic with my high-fat, unhealthy hot dog.

One of our first patients is a man who heard we were on reserve and has walked in to say that he has been having headaches. I pull the blood pressure cuff from the doctor's bag and take his blood pressure. The result: 220/110. This level of hypertension is associated with strokes and is extremely dangerous. I get the man's history—high blood pressure for years, recently ran out of medications. Should we take him to Regina for admission to hospital, or prescribe medication now and hope he doesn't stroke? We present the options to the patient, and he rejects the idea of travelling to hospital. "Been there before. Wasn't treated good. Don't want to go to the city." He is adamant.

There is an oral medication in our medical kit that treats high blood pressure, and we administer it to him on the spot. Within thirty minutes, his BP comes down to an acceptable range. Susanne makes a phone call and arranges for prescription meds for the next day to be sent from the pharmacy in nearby Wynyard. We often use the drugstore's transport service to deliver prescription medications to the reserve. I feel he will be safe.

I spend most of the rest of the day seeing patients by appointment, as I often do. At the end of the clinic day, about 3:30 p.m., we pack up the plastic boxes, the computer, and the files, and don our parkas. It will be dark by the time we get home.

As I mentioned in an earlier chapter, there appears to be a genetic predisposition to diabetes among the Indigenous people of Turtle Island, aggravated by the introduction of industrial foods and sedentary habits. Studies of populations, such as the Pima people (another name for the O'odham Peoples) of the Sonoran Desert, show links to diabetes among those with low levels of physical activity, high-carbohydrate diets, and obesity. A landmark study from the US in the early 1990s looked at genetically identical Indigenous groups, one in Arizona and one in Mexico. The Mexican Pima were found to have diabetes at a rate of 5 percent, while the Arizona Pima had a rate of 34 percent. (For women, the gap was wider, with 8.5 percent in Mexico and 40 percent in Arizona.) The body composition of the

Arizona Pima group showed higher fat mass, lower physical activity, and higher dietary fat intake.[2] From what I have learned from my colleagues, these same factors have influenced rates of diabetes in Indigenous people in Canada.

Roxane Wagner worked with diabetics in the Touchwood Hills communities for several months before she realized that they had lost the ability to cook. They had memories of their parents growing vegetables in their gardens in summer and hunting for wild meat in the hills in the fall; many of those skills, although prevalent for decades after the signing of the treaties, had been lost. The loss of traditional ways, a pillar of Canada's assimilation policy, had brought epidemic disease to reserves where the closest produce market was located in Wynyard (thirty minutes by car) or Regina (two hours). Adopting a factory-made diet had contributed to the skyrocketing presence of diabetes.

Roxane began her work by asking people in her diabetes education classes if they would be interested in fresh vegetables from a garden. By spring the next year, she had hatched a plan and received external funding. With experience in food services administration, Roxane knows how to write a grant application. The provincial Child and Family Services branch agreed to provide $2,000 to support the construction of raised gardens. Roxane created the gardens' design and then bought materials for them from the grant funds. There was enough money left to hire Indigenous construction workers to build raised wooden beds, thirty-two feet by eight feet. After the beds were filled with soil, she bought seeds using program funds. The designing, building, and planting was done in collaboration with the local people.

---

2   Leslie O. Schulz, Peter H. Bennett, Eric Ravussin, Judith R. Kidd, Kenneth K. Kidd, Julian Esparza, and Mauro E. Valencia, "Effects of Traditional and Western Environments on Prevalence of Type 2 Diabetes in Pima Indians in Mexico and the US," *Diabetes Care* 29, no. 8 (August 2006): 1866–1871, https://doi.org/10.2337/dc06-0138.

She reflected, "Everyone was proud of these gardens, but they didn't produce enough to feed the community." The four Touchwood Hills communities applied for a larger grant, and it was funded. As the next spring arrived and summer bloomed, there were grow tunnels behind each health centre on reserve, hidden from the wind and the evaporating effects of the summer sun. They are now producing bushels of vegetables for local consumption on reserve. Roxane, with her Indigenous partners and advocates, continues the grant application process with success, which supports sustainable agriculture and healthy eating on each reserve. Local residents now take the lead in canning classes, hunting preservation classes, and traditional culture classes. Indigenous people here are regaining control of their food environment.

Michelle Archer, a dietitian who shares the Aboriginal Diabetes Initiative work with Roxane on the Touchwood Hills reserves, has a different focus. She is a woman with a large presence and a big heart. Michelle has worked with Indigenous people for many years and is skilled and knowledgeable about the effects of diabetes. She often calls me on my cellphone to discuss the status of individual patients and the need to adjust insulin dosing. I respect her ability to teach carbohydrate counting, to propose changes in treatment, and to involve diabetics in their own care. She also has an A-to-Z knowledge of Ottawa's Non-Insured Health Benefits program, as I learned when I spoke with her about our diabetic patients recently discharged from hospital.

On one of my days on duty at the Regina General, I received a call from the ER physician on duty. I walked down the corridor to the Emergency Room and was introduced to Brian, who had driven in from the Touchwood Hills. He was relatively young at thirty-eight and had lived with diabetes for ten years. He was thin with an athletic build, and had steady employment as a security officer at a mine construction site about an hour from his home on the reserve.

Brian's diabetes required insulin for control, but he had not been following the instructions he received from previous doctors. His three-month blood test, or hemoglobin A1c, an average of the last three months of blood sugar, was 12 percent—more than twice the upper limit of what is regarded as normal. He had lost most of the feeling in his feet (peripheral neuropathy) and developed ulcers on three toes of his right foot. He had never missed a day of work; his wife and two children depended on him. But his foot ulcer had become infected, and he needed admission to hospital for antibiotic treatment.

I consulted a vascular surgeon. After his assessment, the surgeon told me that the fastest way to get Brian back to work would be to amputate the toes. This was a harsh calculation: without surgery, Brian would need a long course of antibiotics and bedrest. Even with that treatment, he might eventually need an amputation.

Brian would have to decide. I sat at the side of his bed and looked into his sorrowful eyes as I gave him the news. He did not want to be in hospital. He did not want to miss work, he did not want to lose his toes, and he did not want any further suffering from diabetes.

Many Indigenous patients are skilled at detecting inauthentic behaviour, and I held back any hint of false reassurance. Brian had been working with Michelle on reserve. A smart man, he would know that uncontrolled blood sugars can cause peripheral neuropathy and foot ulcers. He had repeatedly skipped appointments with his doctors. I sat with him in silence for a while and then offered empathy. I could not offer more.

The surgery took place the next day. Brian returned to reserve to heal after a few days of recovery, with a promise to see me at an upcoming clinic on reserve near his home.

Two weeks later, I am back on reserve with my colleague Susanne. Brian shows up for his appointment, just before noon, and says he wants to improve his diabetes control. We order him a Libre machine to help him monitor his blood sugars at home without pricking his finger. He is wearing a large plastic boot, an "off-loading" apparatus that allows him to walk without placing pressure on his damaged right foot.

We undress the foot and inspect it for healing. It looks good, and everyone is pleased, especially Brian. He had been eating better, and his glucometer provided evidence that his blood sugars had improved. Keeping the numbers in the normal range requires diligence, and I am sure the Libre will help him. He had been doing a good job; he just needed some tweaks in his diabetes management. We adjust his insulin dosing and give him a permission slip to return to work, with accommodations for his walking boot.

It has been a long morning; Susanne and I take a break for lunch. We have brought our own meals from home, and we join Michelle Archer at a table in the lunchroom where she sits with a plastic Tupperware container filled with leftovers that she has heated in the microwave. Still thinking about Brian, I tell Michelle that I'm perplexed by his history of skipping medication and appointments, given the stakes in his personal life. Wondering how Brian reached the point of amputation, I ask her: Why are these diabetic patients in such poor control? Why do they no-show for their appointments?

Michelle has been working here for a long time and is frustrated with the culture of "noncompliance," a word that is increasingly outmoded, and she does not take poor diabetes control personally.

"One of the major issues is confidentiality," she said. "Everybody is related to someone on reserve. Often there is a relative who works here at the clinic. The diabetics, or anyone else with a chronic condition, may not want to be seen as sick. So they stay away."

Thinking about the abuse of power that occurs in all communities, both settler and Indigenous, she continues: "It gets really nasty around the health centre building at election time. If you're related to somebody who was defeated in the election, all of a sudden you're from the wrong family. You don't feel welcome. The loss of the communal spirit provided by the Elders that was part of traditional Indigenous values is likely a result of colonialism."

She takes a bite of her lunch. "The 8:00 a.m. to 5:00 p.m. hours don't work for some people. Transportation can be a barrier, especially in the winter. We don't have regular doctors. We have to work on building trust with Indigenous patients, piece by piece.

"In the past few years," she continues, "two innovations have improved the quality of diabetes treatment. Both are covered under Canada's Non-Insured Health Benefits for First Nations diabetics. First, a medication called Ozempic has been accepted by the community." Ozempic is the drug name for semaglutide, a GLP-1 (glucagon like peptide 1) for type 2 diabetes. It increases insulin secretion from the pancreas and controls blood sugars. It is injected weekly and is associated with blunting of hunger.

Michelle says, "I've seen real improvement in diabetes control with Ozempic use. People see that their blood sugars are better. They also notice that they are losing weight. Then other people in the community notice that they are looking better. Word of mouth has helped, especially with the men. The talk at the pool hall and on the golf course is about this new injectable.

"The other innovation is the introduction of continuous glucose monitors, or CGMs, that allow patients to avoid the constant pricking of their finger to measure blood sugar." These devices, which use a small electrode placed on the skin, help diabetics track their blood sugar levels.

Michelle continues: "Diabetics can see their blood sugar on a handheld monitor whenever they want. They can see how different foods in a meal change blood sugar so they can adjust their eating habits, and in some cases they allow their physician to modify their insulin dosing."

This is all good news, but one must keep in mind, as the Diabetes Canada Clinical Practice Guidelines points out, that stressors, along with chaotic or overwhelming living conditions, can undermine a person's capacity to cope with and manage their diabetes.[3]

Back in Regina, I am called to the ER and am presented with another diabetic—a twenty-six-year-old Indigenous man who has been transported to the hospital by helicopter with diabetic ketoacidosis. His sister tells me that he stopped taking his insulin six months ago, and his blood sugar is dangerously high. I don't ask why he stopped taking his insulin. The priority is to save his life. The cells of his body have been overwhelmed with sugar and are producing acids in the bloodstream. The acids and the blood sugar are bathing his brain; he is comatose and has entered a dangerous phase. I call out instructions to the nurses around his gurney in the ER. Start fluids, start insulin drip. I pick up the phone and call the Intensive Care Unit physician.

Within hours, we have saved this patient's life. Several days later, out of the ICU and on the ward, he thanks me from his hospital bed. His blood sugar is under control, and he is ready to go home—back to the environment that got him here in the first place. We've learned that his kidneys have failed, so he will have to make regular visits to the hospital for dialysis for the rest of his life. I smile at him, shake his hand, and wish him luck. I wish that I could do more. The next time that I see him, he is on the dialysis shuttle.

Roxane gives me an interesting perspective on the challenges posed by the cost of food. She is very practical. If a food basket for a family of four costs $250 a week, the family will be spending $13,000 per year to eat. That does not include the price of gas for the necessary car trip into the city to get food. If you have three hundred families on reserve, they

---

3   Crowshoe et al., "Type 2 Diabetes and Indigenous Peoples."

would collectively spend $3.9 million on food. If some of that food basket can be procured locally, especially the fresh vegetables, the families won't have to drive to the city as often for groceries. The production of meat is something else. It would require livestock development, or the sharing or sale of local game from hunting expeditions. The reserves are planning to scale up their local food production, with a special interest in sustainable traditional food production. Building grow tunnels has increased awareness among people in the community, with a belief that a change in their food system can occur and vastly improve quality of life on reserve. Workshops are held inside the grow tunnels in a non-threatening environment where community members can actively engage. Conversations about gardening with their grandparents are occurring at community events, at the school, and at unexpected places such as the community gas station or convenience store. The power of physically seeing grow tunnels produce fresh vegetables for the community has changed the conversation and empowered people to take control of their food systems. Reversing the destruction of the traditional lifestyles by the federal government's history of assimilation policies will take time, but I am hopeful.

THE SPIRIT JOURNEY

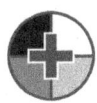

Outside, it is cool and sunny; inside the hospital the ambience is, as always, fluorescent-lit, with that peculiar smell that blends cleaning fluids, cafeteria food, and human distress. Joe is a sixty-four-year-old Indigenous man who has come to the hospital from one of the reserves in southeastern Saskatchewan. He has long grey hair and a slim build that suggests he was a strong, muscular man in the past. His dark eyes have seen the pain that has been visited on his people, and they sparkle with anger.

Diabetes has ravaged his kidneys, and he is on dialysis. Diabetes has also caused peripheral neuropathy, a condition that destroys the nerves, so he has no feeling in his legs. His foot ulcers are open silver-dollar-sized wounds—one on his left ankle, one on the bottom of his right foot. The vertical scar on his chest tells me that he underwent open heart surgery in the past. Undiagnosed heart attacks prior to this surgery damaged his heart muscle, which now only functions at 50 percent of its original capacity. As a result, he suffers from periodic heart failure, a condition where his lungs fill up with thin serous fluid that makes it difficult for him to breathe. His doctors have provided him with a concoction of diuretics to help remove the fluid in the lungs, along with frequent dialysis. Some of the vessels in his legs are blocked; the oxygenated blood flow to his legs is impeded, and he cannot walk across the room. Due to this poor blood flow, the ulcers on his feet have become infected. He has been in the hospital for several weeks, and I have been visiting him daily in his hospital room. The room smells like rotting flesh.

Joe is lying in a bed with antibiotics flowing through an intravenous needle in his left arm. He is staring at the ceiling and does not look at me. His light-haired wife sits at his bedside. I address my questions to Joe, but it is his wife who speaks.

"How are the legs today?"

"The nurses just did the dressing changes," she says.

We spend a few minutes discussing the medical aspects of his hospital stay and then get into the spiritual. I raise the question of end-of-life care.

"I'm really worried that your illness is getting worse."

She responds: "He's a strong man, and he'll survive."

I have long experience in navigating end-of-life conversations. When the patient and their family are in denial, it becomes a dance, not a wrestling match.

"Have you ever thought about what would happen if things don't go the way you want?"

Silence. I am afraid that they will blame the medical system—or me—if Joe's condition worsens. Life would be better if they didn't have to ask for help from the white people who stole the land that belonged to Joe's people, denied them medical care on reserve, and treated them with disrespect. I feel tension in the room and know that only a miracle will return Joe to his home.

"The infection in your legs is a big problem, and the antibiotics we're giving you don't seem to be healing you. Do you mind if I get the cardiovascular surgeon to see you?"

They both nod in agreement.

A few hours later, I'm back. Dr. Kopriva had visited Joe and his wife and explained that the amputation of both legs is the only possible response to Joe's persistent infection. He will be in a wheelchair for the rest of his life. Joe's wife sits quietly, long braid over her right shoulder. She's wearing a flowery skirt, Birkenstock sandals, and a worn T-shirt.

"I understand you met with Dr. Kopriva," I say. "He's a very experienced surgeon."

"Yeah, he wants to cut off my legs." Joe is now speaking, looking directly at me.

"How do you feel about it?"

"I don't want it." He holds my gaze. His wife nods in agreement.

I pause in reflection. After several minutes of uncomfortable silence, I decide that it's my responsibility to raise the subject of death once more.

"You've been in the hospital a long time. As you think about the future, what concerns you the most? What things would you like to avoid?"

I am using the if/then communication style. If the infection does not get better, then what? If he is in a wheelchair, then what? I also think, If his heart stops, then what?

He looks away from me and stares at the wall. He whispers: "I am not entering the Spirit World yet."

With patients from any background, the word *death* is often a conversation-stopper. Patients and visitors use evasive terms instead: pass away, go to Jesus, join the choir, meet their maker. Indigenous people sometimes speak of entering the Spirit World. By some traditional accounts, it takes four days for the spirit to journey to its resting place. When an Indigenous person dies in hospital, it is common for the community to transport their body to their home territory where a traditional wake is organized. From what I have heard, these ceremonies may involve both Christian and Indigenous beliefs in a combination that varies with the family and the community.

With Joe, I have avoided the term *death*, but even so the conversation is stalled. I may have planted the seed for Joe and his wife to consider their options, but I've probably lost my opportunity to establish trust. I get up gently, leave the room, and check my own feelings. I'm suddenly angry. I am frustrated that he and his wife will not let go of their pride and face reality. By some interpretations, to accept one's impending death is to sin against the Christian God. Within the Catholic Church in particular, there is a strong belief that turning off life support is the same as killing. Prolonging life for people who are suffering is seen as the best of care. And when the family will not agree to treatment that relieves pain and suffering, I feel empathy, frustration, and impotence.

Joe is dying, and I am his physician today. As physicians, we are trained to relieve pain and help patients die with grace. However, I know that everyone faces death in different ways. Death is a personal journey, and it is important to allow the patient to follow their own path. My problem is that I do not know where Joe fits on the continuum of Christian-Indigenous beliefs.

David Mandelbaum, a Chicago-based anthropologist who interviewed Saskatchewan Cree in 1935 through '36, wrote that there is a single all-powerful Creator in the Plains Cree belief system.[1] We cannot see the Great Spirit; the spirit powers that we experience are intermediaries between the Great Spirit and mankind. Spirit powers abound everywhere: in animals, birds, trees, stones, and in spirit beings like the Trickster. There is a life force present in all living things; it enters the body at birth and leaves at death. After death, the life force leaves the body and wanders for four days before entering the Spirit World. In the Spirit World, men, women, and children live a carefree life.

---

1   Mandelbaum, *The Plains Cree*.

For Indigenous people, the past experimentation on patients by medical doctors and the trauma from residential schools has resulted in a distrust of the conventional settler medical system. They sometimes reject a prognosis of impending death from a non-Indigenous physician.

As I look in on Joe over the next few days, he continues to avoid the topic of death and the need to prepare. The smell in his room gets stronger as the flesh on his feet and extending up his legs turns from pink to black. The writing is on the wall. He is not going to get better. I speak with a contact in the local university's Indigenous studies faculty about my frustration. She suggests that some Indigenous patients are lost in a negative middle ground; they reject white medicine, but they have been cut off from the traditional wisdom that would lead them home to the Spirit World.

I am a physician serving Indigenous people, but I don't speak any of the languages, and I don't understand the nuances of how spiritual beliefs may change from Nation to Nation. I have only a general idea, supported by some anthropological training before entering medical school decades ago, about spirit powers and the ceremonial aspects of death and dying. I know that Joe will die sooner rather than later, and there is nothing I can do about it. However, I don't know how he is approaching death—whether from a traditional, Christian, or non-believing direction.

My own approach to death has changed with multiple exposures to it as a doctor. When I was a child, I believed in the stereotypical heaven with angels and pearly gates. My experience around death has led me to have a deep respect for the natural process of life's end, and my outlook has become more spiritual. Church was an important part of my childhood, and it continues to be a source of community for me, but I have a skeptical view of organized religion. The mainstream church, in too many cases, embodies individualism, consumerism, and materialism.

For me, Jesus teaches us a social message. As I have explored modern religious writers, I have come to believe that Jesus represents an anti-empire movement. We are called to live in community with others; to live simply, humbly, and justly; and to share love and resources with one another and with all who are in need.[2] I have struggled to give up the rescuer role while learning to communicate with my patients.

It is clear to me that much of European–North American society has rejected the church and we have entered a post-Christian era. Church attendance is dropping, and churches are closing. The trend away from the church seems to be more gradual among my Indigenous patients. The 2021 Statistics Canada National Household Survey reported that 1.8 million people identified as Indigenous, with 53 percent of these identifying as Christian.[3] I recently discovered a story in an old children's book in the basement of my parents' house, a book that was probably used in residential schools. It tells a story, with drawings of a white man with a long black robe sitting with an Indigenous man with braids and a moccasin jacket. The white man describes the life of a baby born a long time ago. This baby had humble beginnings but grew up to become a great chieftain. He became great because of what was in his heart. He didn't own many horses or many bows and arrows. He didn't care about pelts and trade. He wanted men to live in peace with one another, with no war. He was great because he was the son of the Manitou, who created all peoples on the earth. At some point, at the beginning of time, the Holy was broken up into countless sparks, who were scattered throughout the universe. There is a holy spark in everyone and everything. The Holy may speak to you from its many hidden

---

2   Gregory A. Boyd, "Foreword" in Stuart Murray, *The Naked Anabaptist: The Bare Essentials of a Radical Faith* (Harrisonburg, VA: Herald Press, 2015), 8.
3   "Statistics on Indigenous Peoples, 2021," Statistics Canada, https://www.statcan.gc.ca/en/subjects-start/indigenous_peoples.

places at any time. It may be a whisper in your ear, or a whisper in your heart. Life is everywhere, hidden in the most unlikely places.

Some of the nineteenth-century missionaries adapted the Christian view for Indigenous audiences. The relationships of people to Mother Earth, and to Grandmother Moon, and also to plants and animals, were interwoven into Bible stories. Many Indigenous people were indoctrinated and became preachers themselves. As I try to understand the relationship of today's traditional healers with our Wellness Wheel health clinic, I think of the writing of Edward Ahenakew. He was a Cree writer and Anglican cleric who around 1925 wrote "The Stories of Old Keyam," stories from a character based on the Cree icon of the Old Man. These were collected in 1973's *Voices of the Plains Cree*.[4] Ahenakew's text has been studied extensively by Indigenous scholars, who conclude that Old Keyam is conflicted, allied both to Cree cultural and political rights and to white standards of success. Late in the story, the character says, "The Indians must be educated to work faithfully with those who mean well, instead of working against them. Appropriate means must be taken to help us see the fallacy of the old ideas on one hand, and on the other the efficacy of the white man's methods in simple principles."[5] This is a controversial statement; we know that Indigenous people have responded differently to the white man's story with a wide diversity of acceptance and denial.

+ + +

At the end of my rotation as ward internist, a colleague takes over Joe's care. I do not feel vindictive, nor wish death on him. I leave Joe

---

4 A new collection is forthcoming in the summer of 2023.
5 See Deanna Reder, "Understanding Cree Protocol in the Shifting Passages of 'Old Keyam,'" *Studies in Canadian Literature* 31, no. 1 (October 16, 2006): 50–64, https://journals.lib.unb.ca/index.php/SCL/article/view/10199/10547.

to continue his personal journey. A few days later, I hear that he has died. More than my struggle with the cultural and spiritual differences, I have tried to understand his struggle with accepting the inevitable. I wanted to say to him: Trust me, I am the doctor; I want to be trusted. But the baggage got in the way, creating an abyss in our communication. His distrust of me made me feel powerless.

When working with Indigenous patients who are approaching the end of life, I often find a mix of Christianity, traditional beliefs, and distrust of Western medicine. I have been trained to speak about death, but the conversation becomes difficult when there are cultural barriers about spirituality, as well as a lack of trust. I am left with an overwhelming sense of powerlessness. The road to reconciliation is messy.

TEN TO FIFTEEN PERCENT

In 2019 I made a final effort to persuade the health manager for the Touchwood Agency Tribal Council to integrate Wellness Wheel's on-reserve medical records with our in-town records.[1] If medical teams at Regina General could review a status report on each patient as they entered hospital, it would reduce the time those patients spent waiting in the ER and provide better care. Val Desjarlais continued to block support of this proposal, as she had before. After four years of working with Wellness Wheel, Val's official position—probably based on discussions with her tribal council leadership—was one of unshakeable suspicions about settler health care professionals and our connections with the Saskatchewan Health Authority.

I was sitting with Val in the Tribal Council office building, which lies north of Highway 16 outside the town limits of Punnichy. It was

---

[1] P. Di Giacomo, Fabrizio L. Ricci, and Leonardo Bocchi, "Integrated electronic health records management system," *Studies in Health Technology and Informatics* 121 (2006): 228–241, https://pubmed.ncbi.nlm.nih.gov/17095822/.

January in Saskatchewan, and I had dressed in layers for the cold: long underwear under my jeans, a cotton turtleneck under a wool sweater, and two pairs of socks. I had folded my down jacket across my lap, and then laid it on the floor. The building was hot, and I began to undress, layer by layer. I wondered again about the contrast with earlier days when there was no central heating, no electricity for lighting or computers, and heat was produced with firewood. As I unbuttoned my sweater and imagined myself sitting in a tent on frozen ground, I was also trying to persuade Val that my data-sharing proposition would save lives through better care in hospital and better follow-up care after patients returned home to community.

Val responded with her usual calmness. She said it was a great idea to follow up with patients on reserve and to create continuity in medical care. She indicated that she had read my proposal and had shared it with health directors on nearby reserves. She was respectful of the work that we do, and I had learned enough about circular conversation to let her talk.

She told me about the close relationships she had with the people on her reserves. She reminded me of the work she had done, travelling to conferences and workshops, to learn about Indigenous health and social issues. And she reminded me that in a multi-reserve community of two thousand people, we had to keep medical treatment confidential. People on the reserve talk. They know who is struggling. We have to be careful about sharing information.

Wellness Wheel's work plan was expanding, covering HIV infection, Hep C infection, diabetes, heart disease, congestive heart failure, kidney health, and more. I reiterated that we wanted to link health care resources in Regina with services in Indigenous communities. Val replied again that she and others within the tribal council were opposed to sharing information. She suggested that the database at the hospital could be used against them. Perhaps someone might share information inappropriately. She redirected me to the principles of Indigenous ownership, control, access, and possession of data.[2]

I had come to a dead end—the legacy of a lack of trust. For over a century, Canadian governments had disregarded the treaties, selling off reserve land while disqualifying Peoples councils from taking part in business enterprises. With people like Val in charge, local governance had succeeded—with painful slowness—in achieving a measure of self-control. She and her colleagues were reluctant to sign over their health data to improve the flow of patient information between information systems on reserve and in Regina. Doing so would open up questions about the use of public funding from the provincial Medicare budget for the treatment of Indigenous patients in the hospital. They feared discrimination. They feared that the health problems of individuals, a sensitive topic, would be shared and become known across the community.

I acknowledged Val's perspective. She spoke again about what a great job the city doctors were doing with our clinics on reserve. By now it was 4:00 p.m., and the sun was sinking low to the horizon outside Val's window, framing her in a silhouette. I needed to get moving, to drive the two hours back to Regina. I buttoned my sweater, stood up, and put on my jacket, hat, and mitts.

Val's work as health manager supported us in many ways. For example, she used TATC funding to authorize the purchase of two computers with printers in 2019. At the same time, she made it clear that the Saskatchewan Health Authority did not own the computers or the data they contained. We hired a private company to install an electronic medical system (EMR) for use at the on-reserve clinics; we then assigned a couple of data entry assistants to input Wellness Wheel data from the

---

2   First Nations Centre, *OCAP: Ownership, Control, Access and Possession. Sanctioned by the First Nations Information Governance Committee*, Assembly of First Nations. Ottawa: National Aboriginal Health Organization, 2007.

paper charts that were previously collected in shopping bags. We could now find our patient records quickly and look back on prior visits with our team.

The learning curve associated with setting up the new digital system was significant—in figuring out how to enter the data and then learning how to use it. The effort paid off, especially when patients' lab results were merged with the EMR. Consults with specialists were scanned in and made available to the family docs. X-ray results and medication history popped up with one click. We had to educate every physician and nurse to create a visit note summing up each patient's symptoms and the treatment offered. These notes are essential to our communication with each other. Since all of us use electronic medical records in our "other" jobs, we recognized the value of quick access to medical data. We also had to respect the reality that the Wellness Wheel EMR was separate from the systems we used at other Regina clinical sites. Val's directive was clear.

Even with the new computers, we were still tied for a time to a cumbersome system of faxing prescriptions. We would type the prescription into a form and print it off. Staff at the reserve clinic would fax it to the pharmacy of the patient's choice. In most cases, this was the pharmacy in the town of Wynyard, which is close by and provides excellent service. They delivered boxes of previously ordered medications to the reserves once a week (although for security reasons, they did not deliver narcotics). For patients without transportation, the delivery of medications for heart problems, diabetes, and high blood pressure was essential.

With the onset of the COVID-19 pandemic in 2020, procedures in the medical and pharmaceutical industries changed. Virtual care visits became the norm, and pharmacies moved to electronic faxing through the computer. Setting up the e-fax system for medication management required collaboration between the EMR contractor and the phone company and happened within a month.

Throughout the pandemic, Wellness Wheel continued to expand. By the end of 2021, the program had moved well beyond the Touchwood Hills. We were active in the Qu'Appelle Valley and the east and north of Saskatoon for a total of nineteen reserves. We started in 2015 with a first-year budget of $45,000. Through the accumulation of bits and pieces, we grew over time to an estimated budget (not real, but estimated from the volunteer hours that we had all been contributing to Wellness Wheel) of approximately $1.8 million in 2021, most of it cobbled together from travel stipends, federal grants, volunteer time, and in-kind personal contributions. The level of support from Indigenous Services Canada was significant. It supported public health initiatives to fill gaps in areas such as home care, addictions treatment, and blood testing to screen for HIV, Hepatitis C, and syphilis. The provincial government also contributed salary support for one full-time nursing position through the Saskatchewan Health Authority and allowed two additional nursing positions with deficit funding. These deficit-funded positions are not committed positions in the block grant funding from Ministry of Health, so they provide no job security for those excellent nurses who work with us. We now have ten part-time family physicians and a central office in Regina. We are conducting ongoing qualitative and quantitative research as part of the team's work. Clinics provide primary and specialist care on a biweekly to monthly basis on each reserve to maximize the value of each visit and to reduce patient travel.

The individual patient is at the core of our care model. Patients are "met where they are," recognizing that their control over their circumstances is often limited. Our in-care and treatment plans recognize the stages of change model[3]—also known as the transtheoretical

---

3 See, for example, "Stages of Change Model (Transtheoretical Model)," Rural Health Information Hub, www.ruralhealthinfo.org/toolkits/health-promotion/2/theories-and-models/stages-of-change.

model, a process of behavioural change that occurs in stages—where even the most willing patient may be slow to take charge of their health. We account for the fact that poverty and addictions are social determinants.

Val Desjarlais, the first Indigenous person to guide Wellness Wheel on a Saskatchewan reserve, died in 2021. After being ill for a period in her home community, she came to Regina, where I arranged her admission to the Pasqua Hospital. When she realized that the end was near, she went home to participate in traditional medicine treatments. I did not see her again, but she is often remembered for her advocacy at many of the meetings I attend. Val was unhappy with her diagnosis, her course of medical treatment, and her doctors, including me—and she told me so. I was never able to build trust with her or have her see me as a fellow advocate.

One day in late August 2020, a few months after the start of the pandemic, I drove from Regina to Day Star reserve with a Wellness Wheel nurse named Vicki. As we passed by the convenience store at the entrance to the reserve, we noticed RCMP vehicles parked on the road—yellow tape draped across the store's front door. Upon arrival at the health clinic we asked the receptionist if she knew what was going on.

She answered matter-of-factly: "There was a break-in last night. All the cigarettes and cans of pop were stolen. Luckily, the store manager emptied the till before he left, so the cash was in the safe here at the band office. The cops are investigating."

We carry our plastic travelling boxes of equipment into the exam room. The home care nurse enters the room and says, "There's a young girl with a newborn baby boy. Can we put her on your list for today?"

I hesitate. Postnatal care is an area of special skill, outside of my specialty as a doctor of internal medicine who normally treats adults.

"I have to be honest. Infant care is its own field, and I don't have a lot of experience."

The nurse shrugs. "We need to get her in the system so she can have formula for her baby. She doesn't have a treaty card. We'll have to use Jordan's Principle. I can look after the kid. I just need you to fill out a form."

I agree to see her, and the baby.

Jordan's Principle is named for Jordan River Anderson, a young boy from the Norway House Cree Nation in Manitoba. He spent his entire life in hospital, caught in a jurisdictional dispute between the governments of Canada and Manitoba. Neither government would pay for the necessary in-home medical care that he needed to enable his return home to live in his community. He lingered in hospital long after his medical team had recommended discharge, dying in 2005 at the age of five. His case initiated a long legal battle, and in 2016 the Canadian Human Rights Tribunal ruled that the Government of Canada's approach to First Nations children had been discriminatory.

Jordan's Principle guarantees federally funded health care to all First Nations children, regardless of whether they live on or off reserve; for those who live on reserve, it is applied whether or not the child has First Nations status.

By noon, I had seen several adult patients with various complaints: hypertension, headaches, and diabetes. Just before lunch, an eighteen-year-old enters the room with an infant swaddled in a flannel blanket. Sarah arrived on reserve just before giving birth, and she had not lived here before. The baby was delivered with the help of a midwife while the girl was staying at an aunt's house. Her father grew up on a central Saskatchewan reserve but now lives in another province. When Sarah was born, her father did not register her as Indigenous. "Why is that?" I ask. She says she doesn't know, and she says she's not interested in registering. I wonder about the possible reasons: political, economic, identity issues...I don't push the question. Her father may have refused to identify as "Indian"; it may be he didn't want his children to identify as "Indian." Maybe he saw the status card and benefits allowed by the colonial treaties as a form of servitude.

The Indian status card guarantees eligibility for treaty benefits, as specified in one of the many amendments to the 1876 Indian Act.[4] Applicants for the card may be screened through a determination of blood quotient. Recipients of the card gain status as *wards* of the Canadian state, a definition that many people view as synonymous with infantilization.

Among other benefits, treaty status allows access to the Non-Insured Health Benefits (NIHB) program. The NIHB is currently administered by Indigenous Services Canada and covers a list of services not supported by provincial Medicare—including vision care, dental care, medical supplies and equipment, mental health counselling, medical transportation, special-diet foods, and prescription and over-the-counter medications. We make extensive use of the Non-Insured Health Benefits with our clinics associated with Wellness Wheel. The good news for Sarah is that her baby will receive NHIB benefits including baby formula, thanks to Jordan's Principle. I sign the form.

On the highway back to Regina, with the setting sun illuminating the flat prairie, I think again about the barriers that Indigenous people run into when they seek health care and about my evolving role. Sarah's relocation to the reserve was the right tactic, even if her ties to the community were slender. If she had stayed in the city, she might not have qualified for baby formula or other health care supports. Perhaps more important, I know that Sarah's reserve has entered a period of stability and careful government. She will find a network of caring people.

Health researcher Michael Marmot takes a stance on the social determinants of health that reflects my own views: health is holistic, health

---

4   See p. 72, footnote 6.

is income, health is education, and health is socio-economic status.⁵ In the years since my return to Canada, I have paid increasing attention to the roles income, wealth, and education play in keeping people alive. In my opinion, social determinants of health are the subject of Canada's Truth and Reconciliation Commission Call to Action #19: "To establish measurable goals to identify and close the gaps in health outcomes between Aboriginal and non-Aboriginal communities."⁶ Direct experience and research have challenged me to look closely at the real causes of illness. For example, a recent research study states that Western medical care is responsible for preventing only between 10 and 15 percent of deaths.⁷ The rest of human mortality is related to social determinants. I don't want to believe, after forty years as a medical doctor, that my work might be inconsequential; however, these numbers put things in perspective.

---

5   Marmot expresses these views during an interview in Alan R. Weil, "Tackling Social Determinants of Health Around the Globe," *Health Affairs* 39, no. 7 (July 2020), https://doi.org/10.1377/hlthaff.2020.00691.
6   Truth and Reconciliation Commission of Canada, "Truth and Reconciliation Commission of Canada: Calls to Action," 2015, 6–7, https://www.rcaanc-cirnac .gc.ca/eng/1524499024614/1557512659251.
7   J. Michael McGinnis, Pamela Williams-Russo, and James R. Knickman, "The Case for More Active Policy Attention to Health Promotion," *Health Affairs* 21, no. 2 (March/April 2002): 78–93, https://doi.org/10.1377/hlthaff.21.2.78.

THE SERPENT

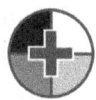

As I write in 2022, the medical, social, and psychological effects of COVID-19 are still unfolding. It has been a strange ride for anyone who works in the health care system.

Authorities have generally described the changes in COVID pandemic patterns as waves—the first wave in spring 2020, the second in November 2020, the third in April 2021, the fourth in September 2021, and the fifth in December 2021, and ongoing.[1] I've sometimes seen the evolution of the pandemic in the form of a serpent, describing humps and dips as it flows through communities over time. The spiritual role of the Serpent is to enter your life and change your focus, similar to the Indigenous Raven character or the Trickster.

COVID, at its inception, was different from the epidemics imposed by European colonizers on Indigenous tribes. It was a global pandemic, and soon after its appearance it affected everyone worldwide, spreading from China to all continents and countries almost overnight. None of us had obvious immunity to this new virus. It affected vulnerable

---

1   Patricia Trebl, "COVID-19 in Canada: How Our Battle to Stop the Pandemic Is Going," *Macleans*, July 15, 2021, https://macleans.ca/society/health/covid-19-in-canada-how-our-battle-against-the-second-wave-is-going/.

populations more readily than healthy and secure populations; very old people, obviously, but also immigrant communities living in close quarters. For the Indigenous people that I work with, it brought disruption in many forms, including but not limited to suicide, homelessness, and a frequent refusal to receive the COVID vaccine—a direct relation to distrust in doctors and experts—once it was available.

The suicide rate has been high among Indigenous people in Canada for many years; between 2011 and 2016, First Nations people experienced 24.3 deaths per 100,000 person-years at risk (time spent during a specified period during which the event at interest could happen to them)—a rate *three times* higher than among non-Indigenous people.[2] The risk of suicide became more acute with the pandemic—the Wellness Wheel network lost several patients to suicide. Lockdowns are not easy, particularly in isolated communities.

One morning at the Regina General Hospital, I meet with a group of doctors to discuss the mental health risks created by the pandemic. As I leave the meeting, my phone dings with a text message. It is a patient on reserve. It says, *I don't care don't call or text me ever*—a simple message, no punctuation, all emotion.

I've heard from Susanne that this man's neighbours are worried about him. He has a history of depression. Nobody has seen him for weeks. He hasn't answered his door, even for the home care nurse, although she could tell he was inside.

Susanne has texted him and received no response. She reached out to me; she knew I had a relationship with this patient. I don't usually share my cellphone number, but several months ago I made an

---

2   Mohan B. Kumar and Michael Tjepkema, "Suicide among First Nations People, Metis and Inuit (2011–2016): Findings from the 2011 Canadian Census Health and Environment Cohort (CanCHEC)," Statistics Canada, June 28, 2019, https://www150.statcan.gc.ca/n1/pub/99-011-x/99-011-x2019001-eng.htm.

exception to this rule. When the patient said he was having suicidal thoughts, I became concerned about what might happen during COVID lockdown. I invited him to call me if he needed someone to talk with. I've heard nothing for months, and recently, at Susanne's prompting, I texted a simple message to his cellphone: "Hi! It's Dr. Boan. How are you doing? I haven't seen you in a while."

Today's response—*I don't care don't call or text me ever*—hits me hard. I've run out of ideas on what we can offer. I'm afraid that he's suicidal, and I want to engage him in care, but I respect his need to be alone. I let it go. As I write this chapter, the patient is still alive, still alone, and still at risk.

From the start of the pandemic in 2020 I have spent time on the COVID medical ward in Regina taking care of settler, Indigenous, and newcomer patients. They were prisoners in their beds, linked to the wall through a lifeline oxygen tube. Each breath is a struggle. Every attempt to get out of bed, every step, causes extreme shortness of breath. As the virus replicates in their bodies and affects their immune response, their lungs are flooded with pneumonia. The very sick patients move to high-flow oxygen, and a pressurized machine is strapped to their nose. No movement. Sitting all day in bed, watching television reruns of *Perry Mason* and *Gilligan's Island*. If their breathing worsens, I call one of the physicians in Intensive Care to advise that we may need to move this patient to ICU soon—that is, if there are any beds in ICU. The COVID death rate per capita in Saskatchewan is one of the highest in Canada.[3]

This failure of my home province to cope has made me wonder about my role as a physician and about the structure of health care delivery in Canada. From childhood, I was wed to the concept of

---

3   James Keller and Carrie Tait, "Prairies Record Country's Highest COVID-19 Death Rates," *The Globe and Mail*, October 11, 2021, https://www.theglobeandmail.com/canada/alberta/article-prairies-record-countrys-highest-covid-19-death-rates/.

Canadian Medicare as a system that provided health care services to everyone, irrespective of age, race, location, or income level. The COVID pandemic shook my faith. I watched as some of my colleagues retired to their home offices rather than choosing to step up to the front lines. I watched other doctors and administrators hoard their resources—concealing the availability of nurses, for example, who should have been available to work in the overcrowded Intensive Care Units. These decisions were related to ego, to budgets, and to the avoidance of accepting the need for change. And to fear.

Resistance to change has always been in the medical system, but it became starkly apparent to me when the system faced COVID. The system was not designed to respond to quick changes. After all, a cruise ship cannot turn on a dime. As a result, many non-COVID-related preventive services were shut down, affecting our Indigenous patients disproportionately. All surgeries, except for emergency surgery and cancer treatment, were cancelled. For a time, there was no community support for diabetics, no pulmonary function tests, no routine cancer screening. Nurses who normally worked in operating rooms, pre-operative assessment clinics, pulmonary rehabilitation, endoscopy, diabetic education, and home care were pulled into COVID-related duties. This left Regina and the smaller communities without the resources to prevent hospitalization, and we saw increasing numbers of very sick patients coming to hospital through the Emergency Room. The non-COVID wards were filled with cases of diabetes out of control, uncontrolled high blood pressure, poorly controlled congestive heart failure, and metastatic cancers. As physicians, we were alarmed by the discontinuation of community resources, but heck—we were in a pandemic and relying on health system leaders and government to work it out.

The fear among both urban and rural Indigenous people was palpable. Chiefs and Elders spoke out and persuaded their members to follow public health measures. Everyone entering and leaving the reserve was stopped at a checkpoint, names were recorded, and the reason to enter or leave the community was questioned. Food hampers were delivered and left on doorsteps, prescriptions were delivered door-to-door, and the movement of Elders from their homes into long-term care facilities was suspended. In the city, it was clear from the start that we were seeing low vaccine uptake in North Central Regina. As Erica Beaudin, the executive director of Regina Treaty/Status Indian Services said, "If you look at the social determinants of health, it doesn't matter if an Indigenous person lives on reserve or off reserve. There are vulnerabilities in terms of health, in terms of standard of living, being part of the community—and perhaps being marginalized within the larger setting." In response, a vaccination promotion program, led by Indigenous Elders who agreed to accept their vaccines to act as role models for their communities, was launched.

A collaboration between Wellness Wheel and Regina Treaty/Status Indian Services (RT/SIS) began administering vaccines at the Gathering Place;[4] the Saskatchewan Health Authority nurses who work with Wellness Wheel volunteered to help. The one-storey building that houses the Gathering Place, previously the Regent Park elementary school, has the features of a typical elementary school built circa 1960 with cement blocks and square windows. Now operated by RT/SIS, it is jointly owned by the Touchwood Agency Tribal Council and the File Hills Qu'Appelle Tribal Council. Its mission is to provide services to First Nations people transitioning to and from reserve. Within a year of starting this service, they had a reported a 93 percent uptake of vaccines in the urban Indigenous population over sixty years old.[5]

---

4 Roberta Bell, "Creating a Safe Space for Indigenous Peoples to Get the COVID-19 Vaccine in Regina," Global News, March 19, 2021, https://globalnews.ca/news/7707655/indigenous-peoples-Covid-vaccine-regina/.

5 Conversation with JoLee Sasakamoose, January 9, 2022.

One worldwide response to the pandemic was deliberate shifting to virtual medical visits. Saskatchewan's single-payer insurance system was redesigned so doctors could get paid through new temporary fee codes to connect with patients virtually. The creation of a virtual billing code was a step forward, but it also created some technological problems. With patients in rural areas, the mobile phone connection was often poor quality, and patients sometimes ran out of minutes on their phones. When I could get through, phone calls were interrupted by children or family members in the household. And finally, aside from these technical complications, many of the conversations were unsatisfactory.

I had a patient with congestive heart failure who told me everything was fine. Then, at the end of the phone call, she added that the swelling of her legs didn't bother her. Swollen legs? A very clear indicator that everything is not fine and only mentioned in passing. A diabetic patient told me that all blood sugars were normal. "When was the last time you checked your blood sugar?" I asked. Two weeks ago was the answer. In many cases, the telephone by itself was simply not enough to help me assess a patient's physical condition.

I sometimes looked at my colleague Susanne Nicolay and said let's take a chance and drive out to see this patient in person. Everyone was subjected to lockdown restrictions, but Indigenous patients were at high risk. Not because they were excluded from making phone calls, but because they often struggled with navigating a health care system that was inaccessible. I spent considerable time making arrangements for procedures on an emergency basis, and I managed to recruit my subspecialist colleagues to preferentially accept these patients into their offices or the hospital. Susanne and the other nurses helped by making sure the patients got to these coveted appointments on time. It was a team effort, and it was time consuming.

When we visited the reserve, our names and the purpose of our visit were recorded at an entrance checkpoint as we entered. We masked all day. All patients were masked. We wiped down chairs and equipment with disinfectant after each visit, since the initial public health messaging focused on the belief that surface transmission played a bigger role than it actually did. I managed to get several patients' delayed surgeries accomplished during this valley of the serpent, which was prior to the ICU crisis. Our medicine chest included swabs for PCR COVID testing that we took back to the Regina lab at the end of the day.

On one visit I reconnected with Bill, the man whose daughter got mixed up with gangs in Regina. As he entered the exam room, I could see that his dress and demeanour had changed. He appeared dishevelled and depressed. His blood pressure was under control with the medication I had prescribed, but his mood had changed. I asked him what happened.

"The RCMP got into the picture. They sent in patrols and ran the gang off. I don't need to sleep with a shotgun under my bed." I'm relieved to hear this, since the danger of children finding a loaded shotgun is concerning for any physician; in fact, it is a major cause of pediatric deaths. He looks down and tears begin to flow. "My daughter overdosed at home two weeks ago. We found her asleep and couldn't wake her up. We tried the Narcan kit, but she was gone. We found needles in her bed. We had a wake and funeral last week. Those kids of hers are so confused. I don't think she meant to leave us; I think it was the fentanyl, and she overdosed by accident." He looks up at me with his face disfigured with pain. I express sorrow. I sit quietly until he composes himself and gives me a hug when he leaves.

The rate of deaths related to fentanyl rose sharply after the start of the pandemic—among Indigenous people, construction workers, recreational drug users, and many people who were simply seeking relief from pain. When Purdue Pharma began marketing OxyContin, a synthetic opioid, in the 1990s, doctors were told that we could treat pain effectively and prescribe it freely. Canadians became the second highest per capita consumers of opioids in the world, after the United States.[6] In 2016, Canada's minister of health Jane Philpott declared the over-use of opioids to be a public health emergency, and the problem deepened with the pandemic. The Saskatchewan Coroner's Service recorded 464 deaths from fentanyl in 2021, compared with 179 in 2019.[7]

The issue, to simplify, is that when opioids were introduced, many doctors prescribed them liberally and too many patients became addicted; if the doctor cut off the prescription, the patient often found an underground source. The illegal traffic in mainstream manufactured drugs became big business. Purdue and its owners faced accusations that they covered up the risk of addiction and ignored illegal trafficking. To date, Purdue Pharma has faced more than 2,900 lawsuits from individuals, hospitals, state governments, and American Indian tribes. In just one of these cases, in February 2022, US courts awarded $590 million to US Indian tribes to support the treatment of addiction and overdose prevention.[8] In Canada, class action lawsuits against Purdue Pharma Canada are proceeding.

With big pharma on the ropes, fentanyl emerged as the dominant opioid in the underground market. Synthetically produced, it is a hundred times more potent than morphine. Two milligrams of fentanyl are often enough to cause death. Ben Westhoff's book *Fentanyl, Inc.* claims that labs in China and Mexico are producing large volumes of synthetic

---

6   "Government of Canada Actions on Opioids: 2016 and 2017," Government of Canada, February 14, 2022, https://www.canada.ca/en/health-canada/services/publications/healthy-living/actions-opioids-2016-2017.html.
7   Nathaniel Dove, "Saskatchewan Sees Another Record Year for Overdose Deaths," Global News, January 11, 2022, https://globalnews.ca/news/8504653/saskatchewan-record-year-overdose-deaths-2021/.
8   Associated Press in Cleveland, Ohio, "Native American Tribes Reach $590m Settlements over Opioids Devastation," *The Guardian*, February 1, 2022, https://www.theguardian.com/us-news/2022/feb/01/native-american-tribes-opioids-settlements-590m.

fentanyl for distribution.[9] Distribution involves a loosely connected ecosystem of independent brokers, truckers, packagers, pilots, drivers, farmers, restaurants, and used car lots. Even as the COVID pandemic disrupted the supply lines for groceries, furniture, and cars, the supply chain for fentanyl survived and flourished. As fentanyl was mixed with street drugs, the potency of the usual mixture of narcotics increased, and so did the death rate.

According to the Canadian Centre on Substance Use and Addiction, 96 percent of opioid deaths are accidental.[10] My colleagues and I have never seen a wave of drug-related fatalities on anything like this scale. In the past, veteran drug users have normally been able to guess at a safe dose, but with the addition of fentanyl into the mix, the reliability of those guesses has gone out the window. In the new normal, users gather in twos and threes to take their drugs and keep their Narcan kits close by, and still they die. Factors that have contributed to the death rate during the pandemic include the lockdown of rehabilitation centres, social isolation related to general public health restrictions, and the diversion of people from addictions support to the COVID-19 labour pool. Bill's daughter was one of many affected by the opioid epidemic. We receive calls from our connections on reserve every week, often with the report of another overdose death.

Among public health experts, the preferred strategy for addressing the fentanyl crisis is captured under the term *harm reduction*. Among other measures, this would provide a safe supply of drugs to people with substance use disorder during their term of treatment. Unfortunately, people who use drugs are often viewed as moral outcasts by many

---

9   Ben Westhoff, *Fentanyl, Inc.: How Rogue Chemists Are Creating the Deadliest Wave of the Opioid Epidemic* (New York: Atlantic Monthly Press, 2019).
10 "Canada's Opioid Crisis: What You Should Know," Canadian Centre on Substance Use and Addiction, 2021, https://www.ccsa.ca/sites/default/files/2021-06/CCSA-Canada-Opioid-Crisis-What-You-Should-Know-Poster-2021-en.pdf.

voters on the conservative side of the political spectrum. Any program that carries the label *harm reduction* will struggle for funding in a jurisdiction where conservatives dominate, as they do in Saskatchewan.

The most important aspect of harm reduction, in fact, is the personal support that is provided to people who use drugs. A harm reduction program, as delivered by a multidisciplinary specialist health care team, is intended to protect drug users from contaminated drug supplies as well as from HIV and Hepatitis C infections. The ultimate goal, however, is to help the person who uses drugs to address their addiction. During the late 1980s, Canada joined a few other countries in pioneering harm reduction approaches in response to rising rates of HIV. It is now common for public health agencies to fund needle exchange programs that provide clean implements for injecting drugs.

Wellness Wheel staff carry plastic containers for the disposal of needles and a supply of clean needles as part of our medicine chest. After we have finished a clinic for the day, we often stop by the homes of people who use drugs, leaving supplies outside or inside the front door. There is also an SHA funded program in the city that allows people to drop by for clean needles.

A supervised consumption site, an environment where users can inject or swallow drugs under the supervision of medical professionals, is much less common. This is a tool that was actively discouraged by some government officials who apparently believe it is better for some people who use drugs to die rather than have safe access to drugs. I say "some" people because a double standard exists. If a son or a daughter of a white middle-class person uses opioids under a medical prescription and gets into serious trouble with addiction, their condition is rightly seen as a health problem, and they are offered a structured course of treatment that may include continued controlled tapering of the opioid use.

Loss of income and lack of social supports led to an increase in homelessness during the first two years of the pandemic. Indigenous community groups were spurred into action by a sense of outrage and concern. From March 2020 until March 2022, a group of hotel rooms were rented for the homeless with COVID. This initiative was co-led by the Saskatchewan Public Safety Agency (logistics) and SHA (health care services), and included partnerships with the Ministry of Health, the Ministry of Social Services, municipalities, First Nations and Métis leaders and organizations, and the federal government. These rooms provided an assisted self-isolation site for homeless people who had no place to isolate after they became infected, or for those who lived in such close quarters that isolation was impossible. Isolation of those infected was a means of keeping the stubborn virus controlled, although it would eventually become clear that a few rooms paid for in a hotel would not be enough. When Premier Moe announced the end of COVID funding in March 2022 with the "Living with COVID" plan, the hotel was shuttered for the homeless, leaving them with nowhere to go.

The conservative Saskatchewan government had announced prior to the COVID-19 pandemic that it would redesign the income support program for vulnerable populations to avoid dependency—that is, to reduce the number of people on welfare by making them more self-sufficient. They called it the war on poverty.

The new Saskatchewan Income Support program was finally implemented in summer 2021 when COVID cases were low and government officials thought we had the virus beat. Among other features, the program changed the design of housing supports. Instead of paying landlords directly for rent, payment would be made directly to the recipients. The thinking was that this would allow people to manage their own money.

"Clients on the Saskatchewan Income Support program are responsible for paying their rent, security deposits and utilities directly to landlords and utility companies, just like any other citizen," said Doris Morrow, the ministry's executive director of income assistance program design. "The new program will help people who are on income assistance overcome challenges, earn more income, become more self-sufficient and start a career or participate in their communities."[11] The new program put the costs of rent, utilities, taxes, and all other home-related costs under a shelter benefit, meaning a single adult would have to pay for all such costs with $575 per month. Clients would receive only $285 to meet all other basic needs, including food, transportation, clothing, and personal hygiene items.

Predictably, the welfare clients found they did not have enough money to make ends meet, and landlords soon began to evict their tenants. For the provincial and city governments, it meant an increase in costs in dealing with the homeless.

We heard about our patients living in back alleys in Regina and sleeping on cardboard. As the weather got colder, the need for action was glaring. A tent city was established in Regina on October 7, 2021, and eventually named Camp Hope. Social service organizations mobilized and collaborated to provide care. Susanne and other nurses from Wellness Wheel volunteered to do COVID testing and administer vaccines. They were known and trusted by the population and were able to provide the necessary supports to prevent an outbreak of COVID. The weather cooperated; it was an unusually warm October.

The camp population included people who used drugs, and a needle exchange was established to prevent the transmission of HIV and Hep C. Over two thousand Narcan kits were used in a one-month period to revive people who were suffering drug overdoses. Unfortunately, Narcan was ineffective against the latest drug to hit the market, a mix of "blue fentanyl" and benzodiazepines. "Benzos" cause

---

11 Francois Biber, "Saskatoon Protesters Take Aim at Provincial Government's Social Assistance Changes," CTV News, October 27, 2021, https://saskatoon.ctvnews.ca/saskatoon-protesters-take-aim-at-provincial-government-s-social-assistance-changes-1.5640838.

slurred speech, lack of coordination, sleepiness, physical weakness, and, most importantly, respiratory depression. There were deaths. The tent city mourned.

One bright fall day, I went to visit. There was a volunteer-staffed central tent with a warming fire and a table set with a coffee urn and snacks. There were bags of food, clothing, blankets, and small tents. There were forty small tents scattered around Pepsi Park near the Regina General Hospital, with people sitting on blankets or plastic chairs. The atmosphere was sedate and calm. Everyone seemed to be smoking cigarettes. Against the fence at the back of the tent city I saw an abandoned baby stroller, and I wondered about the pregnant women with HIV that were no doubt living at Camp Hope. With daily medication, their risk of transmitting HIV to their baby can be less than 1 percent, but without the medication their children would require HIV medication for life. The current estimated lifetime cost of HIV medication is $1.2 million per child. Wouldn't it make sense to invest in resources to prevent HIV transmission in these women? Or to provide safe injection sites, so they wouldn't have to use contaminated needles?

I wondered, too, about the prevalence of syphilis, especially among the homeless. This was an issue that nobody wanted to consider. On the reserve, Wellness Wheel had started talking to patients about syphilis as part of our core package of services, and we were conducting frequent testing. In the city, with the news media and the health system focused on COVID prevention and vaccines, few people thought to get tested for sexually transmitted infections. Further, syphilis had a stigma attached, as a disease associated with promiscuity, dementia, and the homeless. The public health agency recognized an epidemic, but it didn't have the resources to do contact tracing. In other words, they weren't able to measure the extent of the syphilis epidemic or to slow it down. Public health nurses were busy doing contact tracing for COVID—something that I believe could have been delegated to a different occupational group. Law students and medical students, for example, are trained to ask questions and could have made excellent contact tracers.

Soon after the launch of the Regina tent city, I arranged a lunch date with a senior elected member of the current Saskatchewan government. I asked her about the redesign of housing and welfare allowances and said that it was having the effect of throwing people into the streets. She said, "These changes were put in place to stop dependency on government."

I asked, "How does a bureaucratic change teach people how to open a bank account? You need a fixed address for that. How does it teach them to balance a cheque book? A lot of these people are living in a cash-only world. How can you possibly foster independence without first teaching life and occupational skills and providing community-based substance abuse treatment?"

She replied, "They're drug addicts, and we can't keep supporting their habit." This is an economic decision, not one rooted in public health. I let it drop and changed the subject. Despite the glorious fall sunlight, my mood was dark. I considered inviting her to join me at the tent city to meet homeless people, but knew it was an unrealistic idea. She knew who had elected her, and abandoning her conservative electorate's misguided views on addictions was not on her agenda.

Snow arrived and temperatures plummeted. The tent city was cleared; I was told that the residents were moved to a warehouse near the railway tracks. If that was true, it meant that they were in from the cold. Nobody in government issued a media release about the cost of the warehouse, its staff, or the cost of feeding its residents. Nobody talked about the cost of the social workers who were assigned to find permanent housing. The Ministry of Social Services quietly rolled back some of the most egregious changes to the Saskatchewan Income Support program, increasing the shelter stipend to $600 and the basic allowance to $315, for a grand total of $915 per month.[12] However, there is still a wait list for transitional housing and related supports for people with addictions, and deaths from overdoses continue at a very high rate.

Through 2021, the opposition to vaccine mandates and COVID restrictions hardened among some segments of the Canadian population. Like many people in the majority who support Canada's public health strategy, I felt outrage at first, tempered increasingly with a kind of numbness and resignation. I had a difficult time feeling or expressing compassion for the unvaccinated people who got sick and came to clog up our hospitals. The deadly virus had mutated to become more infectious, and as time has passed we have learned that it continues to change. The vaccine was one of our primary tools for slowing it down, in addition to other essential public health measures like well-fitting masks and proper ventilation for indoor spaces. The refuseniks were swallowing online disinformation from conspiracy theorists and hate groups. By October, our system was in crisis once again.

Our doctors' group in Regina wrote the provincial Ministry of Health and other authorities to let them know that conditions in the hospital had become desperate. We took to social media and tweeted our concerns. Our beds were full, and there were no more Intensive Care nurses to recruit from anywhere in southern Saskatchewan. ICU nursing is a special skill and requires advanced training and experience. The government was offering pandemic pay to anyone who stepped forward, but we had simply run out of willing, qualified people.

In November, when all the ICU beds were full, Saskatchewan began a program to fly intubated, sedated patients with COVID to other

---

12   On March 23, 2022, the Government of Saskatchewan released its 2022–23 budget, which included the increase to SIS. Nicholas Frew, "'Slap in the Face': $30-a-Month Income Support Increases in Sask. Budget Not Enough, Advocates Say," CBC News, March 23, 2023, https://www.cbc.ca/news/canada/saskatchewan/saskatchewan-budget-income-support-sis-said-1.6787939.

provinces for care. Twenty-seven patients were flown to Ontario at a reported one-way travel cost of $787,532.[13] That is approximately $29,000 per patient for each flight out of Saskatchewan. This figure does not include the cost of treatment in Ontario or the cost of flying the survivors home. I was moved to compare this high cost, the result of official mismanagement, with the government's apparent indifference to the fentanyl crisis.

One of our patients, Joyce from the Touchwood Hills, was unvaccinated despite having been given opportunities to receive the COVID vaccine—she had heard that it made people sick. Despite urging, she still declined vaccination.

One day Joyce found that every breath was an effort. A family member drove her to the closest rural medical facility, where the doctor tested her for COVID. The result was positive. Even with an oxygen mask, she still was not able to breathe. The rural doctor called the COVID hotline, and a helicopter was dispatched to pick her up. She arrived in Regina in very poor condition, and she was sent straight to the ICU. I found her there, sedated, intubated, and with multiple IV bags hanging around her bed. I spoke to the critical care doctor and found out that the ventilator settings were not too high. This was a good sign.

In mid-October Joyce was transported to Ontario. She spent several days in an ICU before her family was flown to see her, their flight funded by the public purse. She lay in a sedated, intubated state for two weeks, after which she began to recover. She was very weak, but she was judged to be well enough to fly back to Regina. The trip, it seems, had changed her mind about vaccination. She now told her daughter Tania, "Tell everybody that you know that hasn't taken the needle, tell them to

---

13   Alec Salum, "Government Charged $787,532 So Far for Out of Province COVID Transfers," *Regina Leader-Post*, December 2, 2021, https://leaderpost.com/news/politics/government-charged-787-532-so-far-for-out-of-province-covid-transfers.

take it now." Joyce's sister and son both got vaccinated, and the vaccination rate improved on the Touchwood Hills reserves.

When I saw Joyce at a Touchwood Hills clinic two weeks after her return, she was healthy, sturdy, and smiling, although she was using a walker. Her lungs had recovered, and she was on the mend. When she told me about the people in her community who had gone for the vaccine after hearing her story, I hugged her. She provided more encouragement for the community than our public service announcements that failed to communicate effectively in a way that would resonate. Her story was powerful, and it has continued to influence many people.

The Canadian medical and health care system has been in trouble for a generation, with an increasing shortage of front-line doctors despite an increasing number of physicians per capita[14] and increasing wait times for surgical procedures and specialist care. Primary care is the foundation of high-functioning health systems. Countries that place a greater emphasis on primary care can have lower overall costs, improve access to more appropriate services, and reduce inequities in a population's overall health. Yet, according to polling released in September 2022, six million Canadians, or 17 percent of the population, are without a family doctor and actively seeking one. That number increases in people who have low incomes and those who live in rural areas. Health human resources challenges are a key part of the problem. Since the onset of the COVID-19 pandemic, family doctors have been retiring or burning out at higher rates, with many choosing to leave established primary care clinics. According to Canadian Doctors for Medicare, one solution is to develop a team of interdisciplinary health professionals, with team members reflecting the needs of the patient population served. Such a model has been shown to

---

14 "A Profile of Physicians in Canada, 2021," Canadian Institute for Health Information, 2021, https://www.cihi.ca/en/a-profile-of-physicians-in-canada-2020.

improve patient outcomes, provider satisfaction, and optimization of scarce health human resources. We need a reorganization of our health care system that fundamentally restructures how medical care is delivered, with a much greater focus on illness prevention, health promotion, and the policies related to addressing the social determinants of health.[15]

In Saskatchewan, the COVID pandemic has brought the system to a precipice, and my interest in caring for patients began to wane in 2020. The effect on me has been a growing resentment about carrying an outsize share of the health care load in the hospital setting. The only thing that kept me going was the prospect of travelling to the reserve and working with Indigenous patients. I began to lose my compassion for others and felt a growing sense of cynicism. I had a keen experience of what's called *moral injury*, a term that often comes up in discussions about physician wellness. Originally, it was used to describe what happens when people are exposed to the violence of the battlefield. It results from witnessing events that transgress deeply held personal values, such as the slaughter of children. What I saw during COVID was a widespread refusal among doctors, nurses, and administrators to accept innovative change, even if it meant saving lives, as well as the exploitation of the pandemic by some doctors in their campaign to profit off our health care system. The health care worker's responsibility to protect and promote health is the foundation of medicine. When our working conditions and professional associates stand in the way of that responsibility, negative feelings flare up.

Canada's Centre of Excellence on Post-Traumatic Stress Disorder has recognized COVID-related moral injury as a syndrome and published a guide for health care workers.[16] It describes symptoms such

---

15   Canadian Doctors for Medicare, https://www.canadiandoctorsformedicare.ca/.
16   "Moral Stress amongst Healthcare Workers During COVID-19: A Guide to Moral...

as guilt, loss of trust, helplessness, worthlessness, and loss of empathy. This resource has helped me to see the distress that I felt after two years of working with COVID as a response to an assault on my moral values, not a sign of personal weakness.

...Injury," Phoenix Australia—Centre for Posttraumatic Mental Health and the Canadian Centre of Excellence—PTSD, 2020, moralinjuryguide.ca.

THE ROAD TO RECONCILIATION

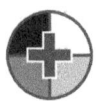

I awake in the night with a vision—a sense that I am both at home in my bed and experiencing another place and time. It is early August and I am lying in a field on a hilltop under the open skies in a sleeping bag in southwestern Saskatchewan. It is a spiritual site near petroglyphs—there are tipi rings on the hills around me—and I am camping on a friend's farm for the weekend. The sky is dark blue, and the stars are starting to fade. It is predawn. There are no sounds; the world is silent. I roll over and face east. Slowly, the horizon begins to glow and the blue on the horizon takes on a reddish hue. A sliver of bright light graces the horizon, and it grows in size as I watch silently. The stars disappear, the sky turns robin's egg blue, and the birds begin to sing. I am at peace.

I see an old brick building in the sky with a long tree-shaded road leading to its entrance. The building emanates peaceful healing energy. There is the smell of sage surrounding it. The entrance is circular and inviting. In my vision, I float inside; without feet touching the ground, I am transported to multiple rooms in the building, each one filled with people—people who look like me, but somehow have no apparent gender and no race. One of the group approaches me with a welcoming smile. I feel a healing spirit, a sense of belonging. These people control their own resources, and they make it work.

During my journey as a doctor in Saskatchewan I have become aware of the concept of intentional whole health system redesign. The pinnacle of health care transformation in Indigenous communities is embodied by one successful example, the Southcentral Foundation's Nuka System of Care in Alaska. A second well-known program in health care reform for North American Indigenous Peoples has grown up in the province of British Columbia with the Indigenous Health Authority. Saskatchewan's Northern Inter-Tribal Health Authority is another example, providing services in a coordinated shared model of care. The Touchwood Agency Tribal Council is actively working with Wellness Wheel to set up a community-based model.

The Cowessess First Nation obtained a transfer of jurisdiction for child welfare in July 2021 with federal funding of $38.2 million over two years. Shortly after this, representatives from Chief Red Bear Children's Lodge contacted Wellness Wheel to provide primary care services on reserve. We negotiated an agreement, but when the payment for travel, nursing support, and physician services was presented, they balked at the cost. As I have explained in this book, transfer of jurisdiction for health care services will require provincial and federal cooperation. With an American Republican–style administration in power in Saskatchewan, it is unlikely to happen. Despite this, we will continue to support Cowessess reserve as a pilot project until we can negotiate full support from government agencies.

Over time through this journey, I have grown increasingly aware of the overt racism in the health care system and, more importantly, of the pervasive subtle racism. I read voraciously to understand Indigenous culture and the background to racism. I talked with people more aware than I am. I learned about two-eyed seeing and stepped into a different reality. I have learned about the treaties and the promise of the medicine chest and what they mean for my Indigenous partners. According to a 2006 resolution passed by the Assembly of First Nations, the treaty right to health is constitutionally protected and includes services that are comprehensive, accessible, portable, and timely, without regard to financial status.[1] This sounds like Tommy Douglas's vision of Medicare for Canada. The AFN goes further to explain that wellness for Indigenous people needs to be approached holistically with a connection to Traditional Knowledge, land, language, culture, and food sovereignty.[2] Canada's First Nations see the treaties as a sacred promise on the part of the Crown, and many don't trust Canada to deliver on that promise. Under colonialism, they have lived under brutal dominance. The dominance and violence have propagated through intergenerational trauma.

Our health care system has adopted a damage-centred approach, focusing on historical exploitation, domination, and residential school trauma to explain poverty, addictions, and poor health. According to Eve Tuck, an Alaskan Indigenous researcher now at the University of Toronto, it needs to be replaced with a desire-based framework—one that focuses on sharing of Indigenous knowledge with a strength-based approach.[3] Indigenous friends have taught me about humility, resilience, wisdom, spirituality, connection to the land, and sharing. As we move forward in treaty, we can learn from each other.

---

[1] Assembly of First Nations (AFN), "Your health benefits: A First Nations guide to accessing non-insured health benefits," 2006, https://www.ntassembly.ca/sites/assembly/files/10-05-20td59-165.pdf.

[2] Aimée Craft and Alice Lebihan, "The Treaty Rights to Health: A Sacred Obligation," National Collaborating Centre for Indigenous Health (NCCIH), 2021, https://www.nccih.ca/Publications/Lists/Publications/Attachments/10361/Treaty-Right-to-Health_EN_Web_2021-02-02.pdf.

[3] Eve Tuck, "Suspending Damage: A Letter to Communities," *Harvard Educational Review* 79, no. 3 (Fall 2009): 409–428, https://pages.ucsd.edu/~rfrank/class_web/ES-114A/Week%204/TuckHEdR79-3.pdf.

Murray Sinclair's statement on reconciliation burns into my psyche: "The road we travel is equal in importance to the destination we seek. There are no shortcuts. When it comes to truth and reconciliation we are forced to go the distance."[4] The settler who seeks to travel this road needs imagination and resilience. Through my own process I have found myself challenged with judgment, anger, outrage, and shame—my own, and that of others. I have had to examine my own relationship with colonialism and privilege, and I continue to work at it every day.

I am constantly learning new things, sometimes in unexpected places. Recently, Stacy Buffalo joined us via online video conferencing to present an overview of Wellness Wheel to the medical students of Saskatchewan. We all spoke to the students for a few minutes, but Stacy's presentation was particularly optimistic. Stacy is the director of health services at Day Star First Nation in the Touchwood Hills. She is a dynamic woman with long black hair and a gentle smile. As she talked about the impact of Wellness Wheel clinics on improving the health of her people on reserve, she praised us. Then she said something that I didn't expect: "Maybe sometime in the near future, we will have our own health authority and control our own resources." She had expressed what I had been thinking, making clear through her statement that we share optimism about the future of Indigenous-led health systems.

+ + +

---

4   This statement from Justice Murray Sinclair, chair of the Truth and Reconciliation Commission of Canada, was delivered to the Canadian Senate Standing Committee on Aboriginal Peoples on September 28, 2010. "Proceedings of the Standing Senate Committee on Aboriginal Peoples," Government of Canada, 35th Parliament, 2nd session, issue no. 1 (Mar. 20/Nov. 5, 1996), https://publications.gc.ca/site/eng/389817/publication.html. Quoted in the Canadian Public Health Association Strategic Plan 2021–2025, https://www.cpha.ca/strategic-plan-2021-2025.

Despite some good news stories, I have become pessimistic about the state of the health care system in Canada. *Emotional labour* is defined as the exasperating burden of being enlightened in a biased society. I feel that I carry an exasperating burden in trying to compensate for what seems to be an increasingly profit-motivated bureaucratic health system that puts middle-class voters and privileged white needs before the needs of all others.

Saskatchewan's Tommy Douglas, whom some label as a democratic socialist, envisioned a country where people might live free of fear and free of crippling medical debts when we become ill.[5] Through his leadership, universal Medicare was established in Canada with health care as a human right. But as neo-liberalism has continued to extend its reach and pushes us backward towards a nineteenth-century version of capitalism, universal access to publicly funded health care in Canada is increasingly threatened. I see profit-driven health care delivery inching its way into the mainstream—a process that supports the wealthy and marginalizes the poor. I also see young medical students with a passion for addressing the social determinants of disease, but who lose their passion when faced with the "business" of medicine. I see average healthy people, Indigenous and settler, wait for access to primary care services even though Canada graduates enough family doctors per capita to serve all Canadians. I am invited to dine at the opulent homes of doctors—homes that could easily house several families. When my hosts express admiration for the work that I do with Wellness Wheel, I thank them with humility and grace while holding my judgment of their display of wealth. These are my colleagues; they

---

5   Tommy Douglas, quoted in Canadian Health Coalition and Canadian Centre for Policy Alternatives, "Completing Tommy's Vision: Next Steps to Expand and Improve Canada's Medicare System," Canadian Health Coalition and CCPA, May 4, 2007, https://www.hsabc.org/webuploads/newsitems/BCHC/Completing_Tommys_Vision.pdf.

all have a heart and passion for medicine, and they respond when I call them for help.

One of my patients in the Touchwood Hills came to the health centre with a present for me. He said he would give me a name: Buffalo Woman. I asked him to explain its meaning. He said that the buffalo woman makes use of all parts of the buffalo to take care of the community. From the hide, she makes moccasins, clothing, or tipi liners. From the meat, she makes pemmican. From the dung, she collects chips as fuel for cooking. From the tallow, she makes soups, candles, and soap. Every part of the buffalo was used in one way or another, and most of the processing was women's work. He looked at me and said, "This name describes you because you take care of our community." In the Seven Sacred Teachings, he said, the buffalo is the symbol of respect.

When I looked up the meaning of Buffalo Power, I discovered that in addition to providing warmth, food, and tools, the buffalo provided a model on how to live. According to the InterTribal Buffalo Council, the buffalo reminds Indigenous people on the plains of how their lives were once lived free and in harmony with nature.[6] I know that this name has not been accorded to me in an Indigenous ceremony, but I am touched by this personal gesture and the respect that my friend accorded to my work with the people in the Touchwood Hills.

I am not Indigenous by culture or identity. I will never become Indigenous, even with the small amount of blood quotient inherited from my mother. But I have been transformed and changed by my interaction with my Indigenous cousins. My learning about Indigenous people has brought me closer to understanding their ways. Their ways

---

6   "Taking Informed Action," InterTribal Buffalo Council, https://americanindian .si.edu/nk360/plains-belonging/itbc#:~:text=%22Critical%20to%20their%20 survival%2C%20bison,and%20in%20harmony%20with%20nature.

are different from my ways; their ways will never be my ways. I have been blessed with the eyes of an immigrant returning to my homeland after many years away. This has given me the ability to view things a little differently perhaps than I might have viewed the surrounding settler culture. I have the stature of the settler class in Saskatchewan with all the trappings of privilege. I have power that comes from the settler class. I recognize that power can be used for advocacy, and I am still trying to figure out how to use this power as an ally of Indigenous people. Then I learn about another of the Seven Sacred Teachings: "Dbaa-dem-diz-win—To accept yourself as a sacred part of Creation is to know humility."

Dexter sits in my private office at the health centre in Touchwood Hills, tall and lanky, almost seventy-four years old. He wears a straw hat, and two grey braids rest on his shoulders. His blue eyes are cool and piercing. He needs a form to be signed by a physician to allow him to renew his licence to drive a school bus on the reserve. It is July, just after a summer rain the night before, and the day is clear, calm, and mellow. We have seen each other many times for minor medical complaints in the past, so we know each other. With each visit, our conversation gets a little deeper.

He has passed his medical exam for the provincial driver's licence. Instead of letting him go, I ask him, "How did you become an Elder in the community?" He bows his head and says: "It is something that happens when you age. People think that you are an Elder."

I persist out of curiosity.

"Don't you get appointed as an Elder, or elected, or anointed?"

He responds, "Well, I found that people just kept coming to me for advice. Nobody gave me a title.

"I learned from the Elders when I was young. I spoke the language with them, and they taught me the traditional ways. Then I went to residential school, then to day school."

"What happened to those traditional learnings while you were at school?"

He says, "I kept them to myself. I hid them inside. I learned to read and write English, but I kept the old language inside me. Each one of us has a spirit. That spirit cannot be extinguished. When I left day school, I went to work in Alberta. The Japanese had vegetable farms where they needed labourers. I worked hard in the fields in the summer and fall. Then I would come back to reserve for the winter."

"And then later you became an Elder. When you were forty, or fifty, or sixty?"

"I got along with people. I saw the good in people, and they started to come to me for advice. I didn't ask for a title. I just kept living my traditional ways. I spoke Cree from my early days, and I learned Saulteaux. I could talk with anyone. I even went to Arizona to give a spiritual name to a Navajo in a ceremony.

"We all have a spirit inside of us. Living a hard life has helped me recognize the spirits. When people die, they go to the Spirit World. If you have not learned to recognize the spirits, you will live in the place of evil. It is a terrible gift I have. To recognize when people are lying, when they are hiding their reality and do not want to face it. I can see it in people, but it is not up to me to reveal it to them, not most of the time."

I feel humbled that Dexter has shared this with me. He would not be speaking this way unless he trusted me to listen. Humility is that paradoxical blessing that you can possess if you believe to the marrow of your bones you do not possess it. The danger is that as you work to achieve humility you may puff up with pride at being humble. It's about being honest with yourself, which is hard. I think about the things that I am hiding and the egoism that has become almost a mandatory tool for me in the competitive world of medicine. I am touched by his simplicity and groundedness.

I am reminded of the Chinese proverb "A journey of a thousand miles begins with a single step." Within the Indigenous community in

Canada, I take hope from the hummingbird. In some Indigenous belief systems, the hummingbird symbolizes courage and determination:

> One day in the forest a fire broke out. All the animals ran, fearing for their lives. Suddenly the wolf saw a little hummingbird head. The wolf asked him what he was doing, and the hummingbird said, "I am flying to the lake to get drops of water to help put out the fire." The wolf laughed at him and said, "You're crazy, you can't put out this fire!" The hummingbird replied, "At least I am doing my part."

I attempt to work together with my Indigenous partners for a greater good. I care. I seek humility. Let us respect each other and embody humility so we can speak to the spirit of the treaties. I am committed to moving forward, to listen to my Indigenous partners and work alongside them to realize goals and a vision that strengthens all cultures.

My vision in the early August morning stays with me—of a healing place that connects the community.

Manacihitowin—let us respect each other.

SEVEN GRANDFATHER TEACHINGS FROM THE ANISHINAABE

- (*Bravery/Courage*) *Aak-de-he-win*—To face life with courage is to know bravery.
- (*Respect*) *Ma-na-ji-win*—To honour all of Creation is to have respect.
- (*Humility*) *Dbaa-dem-diz-win*—To accept yourself as a sacred part of Creation is to know humility.
- (*Truth*) *De-bwe-win*—To know these things is to know the truth.
- (*Honesty*) *Gwe-ya-kwaad-zi-win*—To walk through life with integrity is to know honesty.
- (*Love*) *Zah-gi-di-win*—To know love is to know peace.
- (*Wisdom*) *Nbwaa-ka-win*—To cherish knowledge is to know wisdom.

Source: Treaty One Protection Office, 300-340 Assiniboine Avenue, Winnipeg, Manitoba R3C 0Y1, info@treaty1.com

POSTSCRIPT

The feedback that I have received about this book has been mixed. Some say that it is a valuable addition to the road towards reconciliation. Others who know me say that I am a compassionate, caring physician—something that (unfortunately) is not always true.

One health care specialist who works with Indigenous people in Canada called me brave. I do not consider myself brave. I like to be liked and, as negative reviews came in prior to publication, I became afraid that my written words would be misinterpreted, and then I would not be liked. This realization made me examine the reason why I took on such a complicated topic. I considered throwing the manuscript in the trash. These stories are not mine to tell, I told myself. The development and maintenance of healthy Indigenous Nations is their project, not mine.

Why did I write this book? The Truth and Reconciliation Commission's Calls to Action make specific reference to health care: "In consultation with Aboriginal peoples, ... close the gaps in health outcomes between Aboriginal and non-Aboriginal communities and [sic] address the availability of appropriate health services." This book delves into the health disparities that have resulted from a legacy of colonization and my personal story of stumbling along the path of learning while trying to make a difference.

The first step in decolonization is to frame one's work in the context of oppressive systems and recognize how I am a part of the oppression.

I have described my privilege in this book and the guilt it brings. Once I was able to get past the guilt associated with my privilege, I was able to examine my personal values and begin to ask questions about the world around me. For the most part, the patients described in this book are not real—they are compilations of many different patients with similar stories. Each patient taught me that I was wrong about my assumptions of the causes of their underlying illnesses. I learned the difference between equality and equity. Equality is treating people the same; equity is understanding the degree of fairness and equality in health outcomes.

I learned about imposition of Western frameworks of health onto an Indigenous reality that describes health in another dimension. I learned about cultural appropriation that has happened on both sides as cultures blended. This is difficult to navigate as an outsider. For example, the popular concept of the Medicine Wheel reflects a complex interaction between Western thought and Indigenous culture. Sorting out this interaction required hours of delving into Indigenous spirituality prior to contact, and the gradual blending of cultures.

As I listened to those around me with openness and willingness to really listen, I began to discover that I have agency. To have privilege comes with responsibility to use the power and to put it back into the community. To say nothing when observing injustices means that you are siding with the oppressors. This book attempts to call out inequities.

Epiphany happened along the way. In this book, I discuss social determinants of health as an important part of addressing the inequities in health care delivery both past and present. Then I discovered a new health care framework to close the gap—the political determinants of health. Politicians write policies and policies shape health. Health care policies implemented by federal and provincial governments have an impact on funding programs—everything from epidemics to education and housing. In partnership with Indigenous nations, we need to seek perspectives and ideas to inform policy recommendations. TRC Call to Action 22 requires that we all engage in advocacy, in partnership with Indigenous patients and communities, to gain control over policies that direct health care resources, and to do it in a way that addresses equity. This requires bravery.

—Jarol Boan
January 2024

TRC CALLS TO ACTION ADDRESSED IN *THE MEDICINE CHEST*

18. We call upon the federal, provincial, territorial, and Aboriginal governments to acknowledge that the current state of Aboriginal health in Canada is a direct result of previous Canadian government policies, including residential schools, and to recognize and implement the health care rights of Aboriginal people as identified in international law, constitutional law, and under the Treaties.

19. We call upon the federal government, in consultation with Aboriginal peoples, to establish measurable goals to identify and close the gaps in health outcomes between Aboriginal and non-Aboriginal communities, and to publish annual progress reports and assess long-term trends. Such efforts would focus on indicators such as: infant mortality, maternal health, suicide, mental health, addictions, life expectancy, birth rates, infant and child health issues, chronic disease, illness and injury incidence, and the availability of appropriate health services.

20. In order to address the jurisdictional disputes concerning Aboriginal people who do not reside on reserves, we call upon the

federal government to recognize, respect, and address the distinct health needs of the Métis, Inuit, and off-reserve Aboriginal peoples.

21. We call upon the federal government to provide sustainable funding for existing and new Aboriginal healing centres to address the physical, mental, emotional, and spiritual harms caused by residential schools, and to ensure that the funding of healing centres in Nunavut and the Northwest Territories is a priority.

22. We call upon those who can effect change within the Canadian health care system to recognize the value of Aboriginal healing practices and use them in the treatment of Aboriginal patients in collaboration with Aboriginal healers and Elders where requested by Aboriginal patients.

23. We call upon all levels of government to: *i.* Increase the number of Aboriginal professionals working in the health care field. *ii.* Ensure the retention of Aboriginal health care providers in Aboriginal communities. *iii.* Provide cultural competency training for all health care professionals.

24. We call upon medical and nursing schools in Canada to require all students to take a course dealing with Aboriginal health issues, including the history and legacy of residential schools, the *United Nations Declaration on the Rights of Indigenous Peoples*, Treaties and Aboriginal rights, and Indigenous teachings and practices. This will require skills-based training in intercultural competency, conflict resolution, human rights, and anti-racism.

INDEX

A

Aboriginal Healing Foundation (AHF), 158
access to health care. *See* Indigenous people and access to health care
addictions, and ACE, 170–71
adverse childhood experiences (ACE), 170–71, 208
African Americans, health in inner-city, 68, 69
agents (Indian agents), and pass system, 3, 155
Ahenakew, Edward, 239
Ahtahkakoop (chief), treaty and negotiations, 2–3, 4
Ahtahkakoop Cree Nation
housing issues, 130
visit of S. Skinner and JB, 129, 131, 140
Ahtahkakoop Health Centre, 131, 140
Ahtahkakoop's people, and Treaty 6, 2–3
Ahtahkakoop Sweat Lodge, 144
alcohol
ban on reserves, 155, 156
binge drinking, 156
consumption and impact in Canada, 152–53
doctors' questions, 154
health issues and deaths, 152, 153–54
and liver problems, 150
in settlement of Canada, 151–52
snub and stereotyping of Indigenous people, 149, 156–57
and social conditions and factors, 154, 158
alcohol use disorder, 154
All Nations' Healing Hospital, 62
alternative health practices, 180
Alvin (patient)
ER visit and hospital care, 20–22, 24
relationship with JB, 22–24
American Academy of Communication in Healthcare, and difficult patients, 50
amputations in Indigenous people, 197, 198, 227–28, 235
amygdala, 159, 207
Anderson, Jordan River, 247
Anishinaabe, grandfathers teachings (Seven Sacred Teachings), 276, 277, 281
anxiety
and asthma, 175–76, 177–78
experience of JB, 209–12
lifelong exposure for Indigenous people, 206, 212–13, 220
in patients, 212
technical explanation, 206–7
from trauma of residential schools, 205, 209, 212–13
typical response, 206, 207
See also stress
Archer, Michelle, 226, 228–29

Asiniwasis, Rachel, 89
aspirin, 4, 4n3
Assembly of First Nations, and treaty right to health, 273
asthma, and anxiety, 175-76, 177-78
aurora borealis, 119n7

B
Bacillus Calmette-Guérin vaccine (BCG), 59
bacterial infections to heart and lungs, 100, 102
"bands," terminology in this book, xiv
Beaudin, Erica, 255
benzodiazepines or "benzos," 262-63
Bill (patient)
   daughter's problems, 122, 257
   hypertension, 121-22, 123
binge drinking (or heavy episodic drinking (HED)), 156
Black, Jaime, 107
Boan, Jarol (JB)
   addictions course, 169-70
   arrival and start at Regina Hospital, 9-10, 19-20
   contribution to the community as goal, 19
   custody of own child, 12, 105
   on death, 204, 236, 237, 240
   and dimensions in the universe, 182-83, 186
   father's death, 210-12
   financial struggles as doctor, 11, 12-13
   as general internist, 10, 34
   medical care approach, xiv
   moral injury from COVID, 268, 269
   on organized religion, 237-38
   own family history and Indigenous blood, 35-36
   patient's complaint to and "Patient Service Recovery Letter," 43-44, 51-52
   practice/office in Regina, 9-10, 34, 149
   reporting of doctor, 147, 148
   return to Regina, 7, 8-10, 19, 31, 32
   with senior member of government, 264
   on social determinants of health, 248-49
   as teacher at College of Medicine, 39
   as university student, 114
   work in US, 10-12, 31-32
   youth in Regina, 23
Boan, Jarol, and Indigenous concerns
   activism in 1970s, 114
   awareness of dimensions, 186
   own progress and changes, 186, 188, 200-1
   at powwow, 47-48
   reconciliation journey, 31-32, 272-74, 276-78, 278-79
   self-recognition of problems, 44, 52
   and self-righteous liberalism, 165, 174
   stereotyping and suspicions, 21, 24, 30
   and two-eyed seeing, 53
   vision while in a field, 271-72, 279
   white privilege, 186
brain
   diseases, 29
   stress and anxiety, 159-60, 206-7
Brian (patient), diabetes and foot problem, 226-28
British Columbia, Indigenous Health Authority, 272
buffalo, as symbol, 276
Buffalo, Stacy, 274
Buffalo Woman, as name for JB, 276
"Butterbox Babies" scandal, 215-16

C
CAGE criteria and questionnaire, 154
Call to Action #19 of TRC, 249
Campbell, Alexander, 35
Campbell, Maria, 105
Canada
   creation of Dominion, 27

destruction of Indigenous world view,
    163–65
  See also federal government; health
    care system in Canada; settlers
Canadian Doctors for Medicare, 267
Canadian Human Rights Tribunal, 247
Canadian Medical Association Journal
    (CMAJ), 124, 156–57
chest pains, and heart, 100
Chief Red Bear Children's Lodge, 272
child custody system, 103
children (Indigenous)
  federally funded health care, 247
  removal from home by welfare
    agencies, 186–87
  tuberculosis, 57, 59
  unmarked graves, 213, 214–15
children (white), and rapid investigations,
    215–16
child welfare, and jurisdiction, 187, 272
chronic illnesses
  prevalence and as problem in
    Indigenous people, 68, 69,
    70–71, 192
  reactive approach in Canada, 18n6
Church and Christianity, 214, 236, 237–39
cigarette smoking, 185–86
circular (or circle) thinking of
    Indigenous people, 49, 52, 53
Clark, Megan, 78
Colin (grandfather of JB), 35
College of Medicine, teaching by JB, 39
College of Physicians and Surgeons, and
    harm reduction physicians, 147
colonization. *See* settlers
colourblindness, 51–52
community health nurse (CHN) of
    reserve, and HIV patient, 81
complaint of patient, 43–44, 51–52
confidentiality, as issue on reserves, 82,
    228–29, 242, 243
continuity of care, 92
continuous glucose monitors (CGMS), 229

Courtney, Rosie, 92
COVID pandemic
  contact tracing, 263–64
  cost of inaction, 266
  and fentanyl, 259
  and HIV, 124–25
  and homelessness, 260–61, 262–63
  ICU beds in Saskatchewan, 265–66
  impact, 251–52, 254–56
  and Indigenous people, 254–56, 262,
    266–67
  refusal of innovative change, 254,
    268
  and Regina Hospital, 253, 265
  restrictions at reserve, 256–57
  and Saskatchewan government,
    261–62, 264–66
  vaccination, 255, 262, 265, 266–67
  and Wellness Wheel, 244–45, 255,
    256–57
Cowessess First Nation, 187, 214, 272
Cree Nations Treatment Haven,
    description and treatment
    program, 132–35
Crozier, Carla, 90, 91–92

D
D9S1120 gene, 196
data on patients. *See* medical records
Davis, Wade, 176, 179–80
Day Star reserve, 246
death
  conversations about, 234, 235–36, 237,
    240
  and doctors, 203–4
  and Indigenous people, 203, 204, 205,
    235
  views of JB, 204, 236, 237, 240
death, as word used with patients, 235–36
decolonizing language, 115n5
Dennis (husband of Mavis), 26–27, 29,
    30, 48
Derrick. *See* Sasakamoose, Derrick

Desjarlais, Valerie
   description and background, 76–77
   and diabetes complications, 197, 198
   illness and death, 246
   on medical records sharing, 199, 241–43, 244
   on visiting doctors, 199, 201
   work with Wellness Wheel, 76–77, 78, 80, 82, 91, 92, 243–44
Dexter (patient), 277–78
diabetes
   and amputations, 197, 198, 227–28, 235
   complications, 197, 233–35, 240
   control by patient, 227–30
   description and outcomes, 191–92
   and dialysis, 189–90, 191
   education class in community, 222–23, 225
   focus at Ahtahkakoop Health Centre, 131, 140
   foot problems, 226–28
   genetic predisposition of Indigenous people, 196, 200–202, 224
   and genetics, 194–96, 200–202
   and insulin, 140, 199, 229
   manifestation in Indigenous people, 193–96
   and metformin, 199–200
   mortality and illnesses in Indigenous people, 190–91, 192
   patients at Regina Hospital, 189–90, 226–27, 230, 233–34
   patients in Wellness Wheel, 87–89, 131, 140, 199, 227–28
   rates in Indigenous people, 190, 193, 202
   services on reserves, 192
   and settlement, 193
   shuttle to Regina Hospital, 189–90, 192
   Touchwood Hills reserves visit from Wellness Wheel, 197–202
   treatment innovations, 229
   and tribal way of life, 201, 202
   types 1 and 2, 199, 200, 229
diabetic ketoacidosis, 230
Diagnostic and Statistical Manual of Mental Disorders, 208
dialysis, medical van and room at Regina Hospital, 189–90, 191
dimensions in the universe, 182–83, 186
doctors and physicians
   communication skills, 49–50, 146, 235
   and death, 203–4
   difficult conversations with patients, 49–50
   family doctors, 15, 15n2, 17, 267
   fee-for-service model, 13–15, 17
   financial issues, 11, 12
   gender inequality, 103–4
   good doctor characteristics, 31
   harm reduction physicians, 147–48
   in medical pluralism, 180
   moral injury, 268–69
   patient complaint, 43
   patient experience with, 44
   relationship with patients, 50–51
   self-employment in Canada, 13–14
   shortage impression, 17
   system before Medicare, 14
   trust from patient, 132
   in Wellness Wheel team, 78, 81, 91, 92, 245
Dorothy (patient), on Indian hospitals, 60–61
DOT (directly observed therapy), 63–64
Douglas, Tommy, 275
drug-seekers, in hospitals/ERs, 21
drug use and users
   addiction in patient, 169, 171, 173–74
   codependent addicts, 174
   deaths, 257, 258, 259, 262–63
   gangs and related problems, 122, 257
   harm reduction as strategy, 259–60
   harm reduction physicians, 147–48
   heart problems, 101

and Hepatitis C, 125
and HIV, 85, 123
at hospital and ER, 101-2
and infections, 99, 169
methadone, 133-34, 135, 146, 147-48
needles, 260
occasional use to addiction (example), 132
in patients seen, 99, 102, 132, 144, 146, 169, 171, 173-74
supervised consumption sites, 260
support for, 102
treatment program at Cree Nations Treatment Haven, 132-34
urine screens, 133
drunken Indian myth and problem, 156, 157
Duffy, Patrick, 19
dumpster diving, 70

E
Echaquan, Joyce, 62
Elders, 115, 180, 255, 277-78
electronic medical system (EMR), 243-44
end-of-life conversations, 234, 235-36, 237, 240
end-stage chronic diseases, prevalence in Indigenous people, 69, 70-71
end-stage renal (kidney) disease, Indigenous people vs. non-Indigenous, 192
epidemics for Indigenous people (generally), 64-65, 76, 216
ER (Emergency Room) at Regina Hospital
as busy place, 111-12
drug users in, 101
duties of doctor in charge, 19-20
role in hospitals, 20
See also Regina General Hospital
Ermine, Willie, 52
ethanol, in race and metabolism, 156-57
ethical space, 52

European culture in 1500s, view by Indigenous people, 53-54
executive functions, and brain, 159-60

F
family doctors
fee system in Saskatchewan, 15, 15n2, 17
shortage in Canada, 267
family names, loss of, 3, 4
Favel, John, 35
federal government
access to health care as obligation, 18, 45, 56, 62-63, 72
authority in health on reserves, 62
ban on ceremonial traditions, 184-85
child welfare system of First Nations, 187
class-action lawsuit by former patients of Indian hospitals, 62
jurisdictional dispute with Manitoba on health, 247
medical vans from reserves, 191
money spent in Indigenous health care, 93-94
survey on Indigenous people and health care, 72-73
fentanyl overdoses and deaths, 257-59, 262
Ferguson, Robert George, 58-59
fifth dimension, 182, 186
fight-or-flight response, 206, 207
File Hills First Nation, 59
Final Report of the Truth and Reconciliation Commission of Canada, findings, 37
First Nations
control of child welfare system, 187
data ownership, 90-91
funding from Health Canada, 94-95
health care system in Saskatchewan, 18
principles in treaties, xv n1

First Nations *(continued)*
   terminology in this book, xiv–xv
   See also Indigenous Peoples and communities; individual nations
First Nations Information Governance Centre, 90
first peoples' arrival to the Americas, 195
food
   availability and cost on reserves, 223, 225–26, 230–31
   cooking skills, 225
   cultivation at Touchwood Hills reserves, 28–29, 225–26, 231
   traditional diet, 193–94
foot problem patient, 226–28
Fort Carlton negotiations, 2
Fort Qu'Appelle
   All Nations' Healing Hospital, 62
   Indian hospitals, 58, 60–61, 62
   tuberculosis, sanatorium, and vaccination, 57, 58, 59
Fort Qu'Appelle Indian Hospital, 58
Fort San (sanatorium), 58
fourth dimension (or time), 182, 183
FQHC (Federally Qualified Health Center) in US, 10–11
fur trade period, 27, 35, 36, 106–7, 151

G
gardening at Touchwood Hills reserves, 28–29, 225–26, 231
the Gathering Place, 255
general internist, work description, 10, 34
genetic predisposition to diabetes, 196, 200–2, 224
genetics
   basics of genes, 194
   and diabetes, 194–96, 200–2
genetic testing services, 201–2
George Gordon First Nation community, 47–48

grandfathers teachings from the Anishinaabe (Seven Sacred Teachings), 276, 277, 281
"granny dumping," 30

H
HAART (highly active antiretroviral therapy), 84
Hancock, Trevor, 152
harm reduction for drugs, 147–48, 259–60
Health Canada, funding to First Nations, 94–95
health care system in Canada
   approach for Indigenous people, 273
   description and flaws, 16–18, 18n6
   fees and payment system, 13–15, 17
   inauthentic mannerisms towards Indigenous people, 179
   intentional whole health system redesign, 272
   national hospital insurance, 61, 61n8
   Non-Insured Health Benefits (NIHB), 61–62
   origins, 14–15
   profit-motivated delivery, 275–76
   provision to Indigenous people, 56
   racism in, xiii, 45–46, 51, 272–73
   reorganization model, 267–68
   rural and remote areas, 46
   structural problems, 253–54, 267–68
   vs. US system, 16
health care workers, and moral injury, 268–69
heart
   functioning of, 100
   tricuspid valve infection, 99–100, 102–3
heavy episodic drinking (HED) (or binge drinking), 156
Hepatitis C
   cost of treatment, 141–42
   description and diagnosis, 125, 126–27

liver and liver disease, 140–41, 146–47
rates in Indigenous people, 76, 125–26
in D. Sasakamoose's case, 140, 143, 146
in Saskatchewan, 125–26
testing and treatment, 140–42, 146
high blood pressure (hypertension), 121–22, 123, 224
hip problem and fracture, 113, 116–17, 118, 119
HIV
contact tracing, 85
description, 123–24, 127
disclosure of status, 84, 85
and drug users, 85, 123
as epidemic for Indigenous people in Saskatchewan, 75–76, 82, 123–24
infections in Indigenous people, 64–65, 75–76, 85, 124, 160–61
patients at Wellness Wheel, 81–82
in reserves and rural communities in Saskatchewan, 82, 123, 124
testing, 140
treatment and patients lives, 84, 124, 263
unidentified patients and COVID, 124–25
homelessness, 22, 260–61, 262–64
hospitalizations rates of Indigenous people, 67–69
hospitals
contaminated materials, 80
in early Saskatchewan, 71
racism and abuse towards Indigenous people, 45–46, 60–61
rates and numbers of Indigenous people, 67–68
See also Indian hospitals; Regina General Hospital
houses, on reserves, 222
housing, as issue, 64, 130
Hudson's Bay Company, 27
humility, 278
hummingbird, 279

hypertension (high blood pressure), 121–22, 123, 224

I
ibuprofen, 4
inauthentic mannerisms towards Indigenous people, 179
income support program in Saskatchewan, 261–62, 264–65
"Indian," terminology in this book, xv
Indian Act (1876), 60, 62, 155, 185, 186–87, 248
Indian Affairs (Department), and Indian hospitals, 45, 58
Indian agents, and pass system, 3, 155
Indian Health Regulations (1953), 60
Indian Health Services, and closure of Indian hospitals, 61
Indian hospitals
class-action lawsuit by former patients, 62
closures, 61–62
confinement to, 60
creation and building, 58, 60
description and staff, 45
memories of ex-patients, 60–61
racism and abuse towards Indigenous people, 45, 60, 62
Indian Residential Schools Settlement Agreement, 218
Indian status and card, 247–48
"Indigenous," terminology in this book, xiv–xv
Indigenous Health Authority (British Columbia), 272
Indigenous people and access to health care
barriers, 18
epidemics from social conditions, 64–65
historical issues, 71–72
medical vans, 191
and Medicare, 72
and medicine chest clause, 55, 63

Indigenous people and access to health care *(continued)*
  as obligation of federal government, 18, 45, 56, 62–63, 72
  as problem, 191
  rates of Indigenous people in hospitals, 67–68
  for remote populations, 191
Indigenous people and health care access *(See* Indigenous people and access to health care)
  barriers to health and treatment, 18
  big ideas for change, 130
  distrust of medical system, 234, 237, 240, 241
  health care system approach, 273
  health clinics, 94–95
  health vs. non-Indigenous people, 38, 63, 69
  hospitalizations rates, 67–69
  and jurisdiction, 94, 247
  money spent in Saskatchewan, 93–94
  national survey of federal government, 72–73
  Non-Insured Health Benefits (NIHB), 61–62
  reform examples, 272
  as responsibility of federal government, 18, 45, 56, 62–63, 72
  as separate from non-Indigenous people, 58
  spending in 1946, 60
  streets-to-hospital cycle, 115–16
  treaty right to health, 273
  virtual visits, 256
  See also traditional healing
Indigenous Peoples and communities
  ceremonial traditions ban, 184–85
  city life, 34–35, 164
  collective resilience, 188
  cultural assimilation policies, 209
  death and traditional ways, 203, 204, 235
  deaths, prevalence and forms, 205
  empowerment programs need, 218–19
  "free stuff" and entitlement for, 55
  and homelessness, 260–61
  inauthentic mannerisms towards, 179
  medical experiments on, 157, 237
  middle ground with non-Indigenous people, 38–39
  misguided government policies since treaties, 219
  multiple traumas, 170, 179
  population in Saskatchewan, 67–68
  in prisons, 116
  relationships with all things (wâhkôhtowin), 180
  and religion, 238–39
  self-control and management, 243
  servitude to external conditions, 115–16
  suicides and suicidal patients, 252–53
  violence in people's lives, 164
  wakes, 203, 235
  "white ways" in fur trade, 36
  world view destruction by Canada, 163–65
  See also children (Indigenous); First Nations
Indigenous Services Canada (ISC), 142, 245, 248
Indigenous ways of knowing, and Western thought patterns, 53–54
Indigenous women
  in fur trade, 104–5
  national inquiry, 107
  prostitution, 103, 104, 105, 108
  as second-class citizens, 108
  violence towards, 106–7, 164
infant care, 246–47
infectious diseases brought to Canada, 56
information on patients. *See* medical records
inherited disorders, 196

INR patient, 26
intentional whole health system
    redesign, 272
Internal Medicine at Regina Hospital,
    39, 112

J
jail, patient from, 112–13, 116, 119–20
Jason (patient), condition and at ER,
    175–76, 177–78
JB. *See* Boan, Jarol
Joe (patient)
    diabetes and complications, 233–35,
        239–40
    end-of-life conversations, 234, 235–36,
        237
Jordan's Principle, 247, 248
Joseph, Robert, 156
Joyce (patient), COVID vaccination and
    problems, 266–67
Joyce's Principle, 62

K
Kathleen (patient)
    description and medical exam, 33–34
    ER visits, 33, 39–40
    social factors for youth, 34–35, 40–41
King, Thomas, 114
Kisikaw Piyesis, Margaret, 125
Knowledge Keepers, 180
Konrad, Stephanie, 91
Kopriva, David, 197–98, 202, 235

L
Lafontaine, Tina, 106–7
land acknowledgements, 32
land settlement in prairies, 27–28
leg infection, 20–22, 24
limbic system, 207, 209
linear thinking in West, 49, 52, 53, 183
liver and liver disease, 140–41, 146–47,
    150
liver cirrhosis, 150

liver transplants, 141
Luu, Thanh, 78–79
Lux, Maureen, 57

M
male power, in medical world, 103–4
Mandelbaum, David, 53, 191, 236
Marchildon, Greg, 70–71, 72–73
marketing, and Indigenous symbols, 185
Marmot, Michael, 248
Marshall, Albert, 52–53
Maureen (patient)
    condition and in hospital, 165–66, 168
    description and with JB, 168–69, 171,
        172–73
    drug addiction, 169, 171, 173–74
    treatment on reserve, 171–73
Mavis (patient), ER visit and hospital
    care, 25–27, 29–30
McKay, John, 35
McKay, Mary (married to A. Campbell),
    35
McKay, Mary (married to J. McKay), 35
medical experiments on Indigenous
    people, 157, 237
medical pluralism, 180
medical records
    on-reserve system (EMR), 243–44
    sharing of on-reserve with in-town
        data, 90–91, 199, 241–43, 244
Medicare
    and COVID, 254
    fee-for-service model, 13–15, 17
    and Indigenous people access to
        health care, 72
    origins, 14, 61–62, 275
medicine
    Indigenous meaning, 183
    traditional knowledge, 4
medicine chest
    and access to health care by
        Indigenous people, 55, 63
    as a baseline commitment, 58

medicine chest (continued)
  description, 2
  as empty or filled with horrors, 4–5
  origin as clause, 71
  testing in court, 56
  in Treaty 6 (as clause or promise), 2, 29, 44–45, 55, 63, 71
Medicine Wheel
  description and role, 47, 179, 181–82
  in storytelling, 48–49
  in traditional healing, 179
  in two-eyed seeing frame, 53
  use by JB, 183
metformin, 199–200
methadone, 133–34, 135, 146, 147–48
Métis people, in Saskatchewan, 130–31
Michael (patient)
  condition, 112–13, 116–17, 118, 119
  doctor's work with, 113–14, 115, 116–20
  impressions of and relationship with JB, 114, 115, 116, 118–20
middle ground between Indigenous and non-Indigenous people, 38, 39
middle space, and two-eyed seeing, 52–53
Ministry of Health (Saskatchewan), 15, 15n2, 245, 265
Missing and Murdered Aboriginal Women: A National Operational Overview report, 106, 106n8
"Missing and Murdered Aboriginal Women and Girls in Saskatchewan" fact sheet analysis, 106n9
Missing and Murdered Indigenous Women and Girls, 106–7
Moe, Scott, 261
monias, 165
moral injury, 268–69
Morris, Alexander, and Treaty 6, 2, 4, 45, 71
Morris, John (Elder and patient)
  prescription, 3–4
  story about his name, 1, 3
Morrow, Doris, 261–62

Mrs. D (Indigenous mother), patient complaint to JB, 43–44, 51–52

N
names, loss of, 3, 4
narcotic medicine, dosage, 100
"native girl syndrome" phrase, 108
Natural American Spirit cigarettes, 185
needle exchange and disposal, 260
Nicolay, Susanne
  amputations in Touchwood Hills, 197
  on HIV and HIV work, 84, 85
  and patient giving no response, 252–53
  work during COVID, 256–57, 262
  work with Wellness Wheel, 78, 83, 87, 91, 92, 224, 228
"Noble Indian" term and views on, 114–15, 116
Non-Insured Health Benefits (NIHB), 61–62, 142, 229, 248
non-steroidal anti-inflammatory drugs (NSAIDs), 4n3
non-Treaty Indians, 72n6
North Battleford, Indian hospitals closure, 62
North Central neighbourhood (Regina), 89–90
Northern Inter-Tribal Health Authority, 272
northern lights, 119n7
Northern Saskatchewan, outbreak of tuberculosis in 2021, 64
North West Company, 151
nosebleeds, 150

O
observational distress, and residential schools, 159
OCAP (ownership, control, access, and possession system), 90, 243
opioid agonists (or substitutes), 133–34, 135

opioids, use and deaths in Canada, 257–58, 259
OxyContin, 257
Ozempic (semaglutide), 229

P
Palmater, Pam, 116
Pasqua First Nation, advocacy for medicine chest, 58
Pasqua Hospital, 69
pass system, and Indian agents, 3, 155
patent claims, and cost of medications, 141–42
patient information. *See* medical records
"Patient Service Recovery Letter," 44
patients seen
    Alvin, 20–24
    Bill, 121–22, 123, 257
    Brian, 226–28
    Derrick, 139, 140, 142–43, 144–47
    Dexter, 277–78
    Dorothy, 60–61
    Jason, 175–76, 177–78
    Joe, 233–36, 237, 239–40
    Joyce, 266–67
    Kathleen, 33–35, 39–41
    Maureen, 165–66, 168–69, 171–74
    Mavis, 25–27, 29–30
    Michael, 112–14, 115, 116–20
    Patricia, 99–100, 102–3, 107
    Sylvia, 149–50, 151, 154–55, 158–59, 160–61
    Wanda, 87–88
    Wayne, 131, 132, 135–36
    in Wellness Wheel program, 78–79, 81–82, 87–89, 92–93, 121–23, 131–32, 140, 199, 223–24, 227–28, 247
Patricia (patient)
    children and custody issues, 102–3, 107
    drug use and tricuspid heart valve infection, 99–100, 102–3

Paula (social worker), 172–73
peer-based medical programs, 134
Pfifferling, Dr., 31–32
Philpott, Jane, 258
physicians. *See* doctors and physicians
Pickton, Robert, 106
Pima people of US and Mexico, and diabetes, 224–25
Plains Cree belief system, 236
post-traumatic stress disorder (PTSD), 178, 208, 217–18
powwow, description, 48
prairies, treaties and land settlement, 27–28
Prairie sage, 183, 184
pregnant women, and syphilis, 167–68
primary care, problems in Canada, 267
prostitution, 103, 104, 105–6, 108
provincial or territorial governments, system for fees, 13–14
Public Health Act (1994) of Saskatchewan, and HIV disclosure, 85
Purdue Pharma, 257, 258

Q
Qu'Appelle Valley, tuberculosis, 56, 58

R
racism, in health care, xiii, 45–46, 51, 272–73
red dresses, 107
Reed, Noreen, 131
Regina
    and COVID, 265–66
    description and history, 7–8, 25
    hospital beds and categories of patients, 69
    Indigenous people in, 8–9, 164
    North Central neighbourhood, 89–90
    and origins of health care system, 14–15
    practice/office of JB, 9–10, 34, 149
    tent city, 262–64

Regina *(continued)*
  unmarked graves of Indigenous students, 215
  in youth of JB, 23
Regina General Hospital
  area served, 19
  arrival and first days of JB, 9–10, 19–20
  Christmas Day, 175
  and COVID, 253, 265
  epidemics response, 76
  hospitalization rates of Indigenous people, 68, 69, 101
  Internal Medicine, 39, 112
  on Treaty 4 land, 31
  See also ER (Emergency Room)
Regina Indian Industrial School, 215
Regina Treaty/Status Indian Services (RT/SIS), 255
Regina v. Badger, 63
religion, and apology for residential schools, 213–14
  See also Church and Christianity
reserves
  alcohol consumption and bans, 152, 155, 156
  confidentiality as issue, 82, 228–29, 242, 243
  description as small parcels, 3
  diabetes services, 192
  and epidemics, 76
  federal authority for health, 62
  food availability and cost, 223, 225–26, 230–31
  gangs and related problems, 122, 257
  garbage collection, 79, 80
  health clinics' role, 94–95
  health workers, 86
  HIV, 82, 123, 124
  houses in winter, 222
  loss of community, 163
  medical services program, 74
  opioid agonists, 133–34
  violence in people's lives, 163–64
  See also Touchwood Hills reserves
residential schools
  apology from Churches, 213–14
  as assimilation strategy, 155–56
  breaking of hope for generations, 216–17
  in cultural genocide, 37
  deaths in, 215, 216
  diseases and epidemics, 216
  emotional support, 218, 220
  empowerment programs as solution, 218–19
  financial settlements, 218
  health effects, 220
  ignorance by whites, 37
  impact and trauma, 158, 159, 205, 209, 212–13, 220
  intergenerational effects, 159, 209
  personal experiences at, 136, 209
  and PTSD, 178, 217–18
  traumatic testimony for TRC, 144
  unmarked children's graves, 213, 214–15
resilience and resilience theory, 187–88
Robertson, Lloyd Hawkeye, 181–82
Royal Commission on Aboriginal Peoples, 158

S

Sacred Circle, 47
  See also Medicine Wheel
salicin and salicylic acid, 4n2
sanatoria for tuberculosis, 57
Sarah (medical student), 39–41
Sarah (young mother), 247–48
Sasakamoose, Derrick (patient)
  description and background story, 139, 144–45
  drug use past and methadone treatment, 144, 145–46
  health issues, 142–43, 146–47
  visit to clinic on reserve and Regina office, 140, 142, 143, 145

Sasakamoose, Fred, 136, 138, 144
Sasakamoose, JoLee, 52, 130, 142–43, 144–45
Saskatchewan
   bus system elimination, 46, 191
   and COVID, 252, 256, 261–62, 264–66
   early hospitals, 71
   family doctors, 15, 15n2, 17
   fees system in health, 14–15, 15n2, 17
   fentanyl deaths, 258
   health care system problems, 268
   Hepatitis C, 125–26
   HIV, 65, 75–76, 85, 123–24, 125
   income support program, 261–62, 264–65
   Missing and Murdered Indigenous Women and Girls, 106n9
   money spent on Indigenous health care, 93–94
   origins of health care system, 14–15
   population of Indigenous people, 67–68
   residential schools deaths, 215
   rural and remote health care, 46
   treaties history, 27–28
   tuberculosis, 56, 57, 59, 64
Saskatchewan Anti-Tuberculosis League, 58–59
Saskatchewan eHealth, 87
Saskatchewan Health Authority, 241, 243, 245, 260
Saskatchewan Health Plan, 72, 93
Saskatchewan Income Support program, 261–62, 264–65
Saskatchewan Medical Association, and medical fees system, 14–15
Saskatchewan Medical Services Branch, 81
Saskatchewan Transportation, 46
Scots, in fur trade, 35, 36
Scott, Duncan Campbell, 37
semaglutide (Ozempic), 229
settlers
   alcohol and Indigenous people, 151–52

decolonizing language, 115n5
infectious diseases, 56
negotiations with, 2
and reconciliation, 274
in three-dimensional reality, 182, 183
on Treaty 6 land, 2–3
and tuberculosis, 56–57
Seven Sacred Teachings, 276, 277, 281
sex work, 103, 104, 105–6, 108
Sinclair, Brian, 45
Sinclair, Murray, 36–37, 274
sixth dimension, 182
Skinner, Stuart
   Ahtahkakoop Cree Nation visit, 129, 131, 140
   approach with Indigenous people, 76
   in beginning of Wellness Wheel, 74, 76–77, 108, 129
   description and work with JB, 21, 73, 74
   later work on Wellness Wheel, 90, 91, 203
Smith, Trevis, 84
smudging, 183, 184
social conditions and factors
   and alcohol, 154, 158
   as cause of health problems, 73
   and epidemics in Indigenous people, 64–65
   HIV and Hepatitis C, 127
   for inner-city African Americans, 68
   for young Indigenous people, 34–35, 40–41
social determinants of health
   description and role, 68
   in diagnoses, 94
   and Indigenous people, 73
   views of JB, 248–49
Southcentral Foundation's Nuka System of Care, 272
spine problems, 166, 168
Spirit World, 235, 236, 278
stages of change model, use in Wellness Wheel, 245–46

Staph aureus infection, 119
Steinhauer, Vincent, 216-17
Stewart, Doug, 215
storytelling, Medicine Wheel as "format," 48-49
stress, 121-23, 159-60, 187-88
   See also anxiety; post-traumatic stress disorder (PTSD)
suicides and suicidal patients, 252-53
supervised consumption sites, 260
Supreme Court of Canada, on obligations of federal government, 63
surgical specialists, in health care system, 17
surgical wait-lists in Canada, 17
Susanne. *See* Nicolay, Susanne
sweetgrass, 183, 184
Sylvia (patient)
   as alcoholic and in treatment program, 151, 155
   background and personal life, 149, 158, 159, 160, 161
   at hospital and later visits, 149-50, 151, 154-55, 158-59, 160-61
syphilis, 166-68, 263-64

T
TallBear, Kim, 202
Taylor, Lord, 14
tent city in Regina, 262-64
terminal diseases, rates in Indigenous people, 68
time (as fourth dimension), 182-83
Titameg (Swampy Cree woman), 35
tobacco (*Nicotiana attenuata*), in traditional uses, 184-85
tobacco (*Nicotiana tabacum*), as marketed form, 184, 185-86
Touchwood Agency Tribal Council (TATC), 76-77, 197, 198, 241, 242, 272
Touchwood Hills area, amputations, 197, 198
Touchwood Hills people, 28-29

Touchwood Hills reserves
   and COVID, 256-57, 267
   deaths and wakes, 203
   diabetes on, 197-202
   fresh vegetables from garden, 28-29, 225-26, 231
   prescriptions delivery from outside, 224, 244
   program to bring medical services, 74, 75, 76-77
   reserves included, 77
   See also Day Star reserve; George Gordon First Nation community
Touchwood Hills Tribal Agency, 74
traditional healing
   and allopathic views, 183
   for asthma, 178
   description, 176-77, 178, 180
   integration with Western medicine, 188
   Medicine Wheel in, 179
   plants used, 183-85
   in Saskatchewan, 179, 180
transtheoretical model, use in Wellness Wheel, 245-46
trauma and traumatic factors
   and alcohol use, 154
   impact on health, 220
   medicalization, 205
   and medical practice, 179
   multiple traumas in Indigenous people, 170, 179
   as PTSD, 208
   from residential schools, 158, 159, 205, 209, 212-13, 220
   science of, 178
trauma-informed care, 170, 179
treaties
   health care provision for Indigenous people, 62-63
   history in Saskatchewan, 27-28
   negotiations and medicine chest in, 2

principles of First Nations, xv n1
and right to health, 273
See also individual treaties
Treaty 4, 27–28, 31
Treaty 6
   description and signing, 2–3
   health care for Indigenous people, 55
   health care treaty rights, 61
   medicine chest clause and promise, 2, 29, 44–45, 55, 63, 71
treaty status, 248
tricuspid heart valve infection, 99–100, 102–3
Truth and Reconciliation Commission (TRC), 36, 37, 144, 214, 249
tuberculosis (TB)
   impact on Indigenous people, 56, 57–58, 61, 216
   outbreak in 2021, 64
   situation and cases today, 63–64
   special care centres, 56–57
   treatment, 57, 58–59, 63–64
   vaccination program, 59
Tuck, Eve, 273
turtle, prediction about pale faces, 1–2
Turtle Island, description, 1
two-eyed seeing, as technique, 52–53
type 1 diabetes, 199
type 2 diabetes, 199, 200, 229

U
United States, 16, 68, 69
unmarked children's graves from residential schools, 213, 214–15
unwed mothers scandal, 215–16

V
vaginal bleeding, 78–79
Val. *See* Desjarlais, Valerie
Van Kirk, Sylvia, 104
vulnerable populations, health care in US, 10–11

W
Wagner, Roxane, 222–23, 225–26, 230
Waldram, James, 93
Walker, Connie, 213
Wanda (patient), 87–88
"wascana" and Wascana Creek, 7–8
Wayne (patient)
   description and drug problem, 131, 132
   treatment wish and outcome, 132, 135–36
welfare agencies, removal of children from home, 186–87
Wellness Wheel program
   amputations in Touchwood Hills, 197, 198
   and community-based model of health care at TATC, 272
   community's control of own health, 95, 96
   continuity of care, 92
   and COVID, 244–45, 255, 256–57
   description, start, and development, 74, 75, 77–78, 81, 89
   diabetes education class and discussion group, 197–202, 222–23, 225
   equipment and rooms, 80–81, 86–87
   expansion, 78, 245
   financial aspects, 81, 82, 91, 93, 245
   first meeting, 76–77
   health clinic of reserves, 79–80
   and HIV, 75, 81–82
   impact on communities, 274
   infant care, 246–47
   inner city location, 108
   medical records, 244
   meetings and issues discussed, 89–90
   ministries of federal government, 77
   mission statement, 96–97
   name as "Wellness Wheel," 75
   needles for users, 260
   as not-for-profit, 90
   nursing positions, 78, 245

Wellness Wheel program *(continued)*
   patients in care model, 245–46
   patients on both a reserve and in hospital, 92–93
   patients seen, 78–79, 81–82, 87–89, 92–93, 121–23, 131–32, 140, 199, 223–24, 227–28, 247
   physicians in team, 78, 81, 91, 92, 245
   protection of patient information, 90–91
   relationship with staff of reserves, 80–81, 199
   staff and support system, 78, 89, 91–92, 245
   waste problem, 79–80
Werner, Emmy, 187
Wesley (Maureen's husband), 168–69, 171
Western thought patterns, and Indigenous ways of knowing, 53–54
Westhoff, Ben, 258–59
White, Richard, 38–39
white matter disease, 29
white people, as self-righteous do-gooders, 165
"white ways" and growing up "white," 36, 37
William (adoptive father of JoLee), 144
willows, as source of medicine, 4
winter life in old days, 221–22, 242
women
   in fur trade period, 104–5
   and patriarchy, 99, 103–4
   pregnancy and syphilis, 167–68
   See also Indigenous women
Wong, Alex, 124
World Health Organization, and syphilis, 167

ABOUT THE AUTHOR

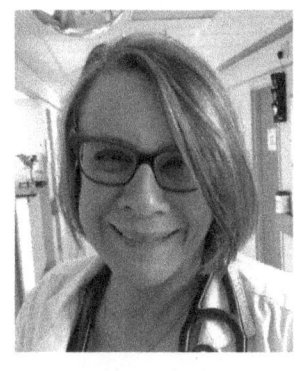

Jarol Boan is a Canadian physician of settler background. Jarol was raised in Regina and spent twenty years in academic institutions in the United States. Upon her return to Saskatchewan in 2011, she became involved in Indigenous health. Her focus on community engagement and listening to ways of knowing integrates appropriate cultural responsiveness between the settler community and Indigenous partners. She is Associate Professor of Medicine at the University of Saskatchewan's College of Medicine, Regina Campus, and currently divides her time between Saskatchewan and Pennsylvania.